# PARAPROFESSIONALS IN THE HUMAN SERVICES

# PARAPROFESSIONALS IN THE HUMAN SERVICES

Edited by
## Stanley S. Robin and
## Morton O. Wagenfeld
**Western Michigan University**

Community Psychology Series, Volume 6
American Psychological Association, Division of
Community Psychology

Series Editor: Bernard Bloom, Ph.D.

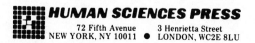 **HUMAN SCIENCES PRESS**
72 Fifth Avenue    3 Henrietta Street
NEW YORK, NY 10011  ●  LONDON, WC2E 8LU

Printed in the United States of America
9 987654321

**Library of Congress Cataloging in Publication Data**

Main entry under title: Paraprofessionals in the human services.

  (Community psychology series; v. 6) Includes index.
  1. Paraprofessionals in social service—
United States—Addresses, essays, lectures.
I.  Robin, Stanley S.  II.  Wagenfeld, Morton O.
III.  Series.
HV91.P37   361.3   LC80-18011
ISBN 0-87705-490-8

THE COMMUNITY PSYCHOLOGY SERIES
SPONSORED by

THE DIVISION OF COMMUNITY PSYCHOLOGY OF THE
AMERICAN PSYCHOLOGICAL ASSOCIATION

The Community Psychology Series has as its central
purpose the building of philosophic, theoretical, scientific
and empirical foundations for action research in the community and in its subsystems, and for education and
training for such action research.

As a publication of the Division of Community Psychology, the series is particularly concerned with the development of community psychology as a sub-area of
psychology. In general, it emphasizes the application and
integration of theories and findings from other areas of
psychology, and in particular the development of community psychology methods, theories, and principles, as
these stem from actual community research and practice.

# Contributors

Sam Alley

Franklyn N. Arnhoff

Judith Blanton

Betty Jane Cleckley

Gloria Doran

Allana Cumming
  Elovson

Alan Gartner

Mary R. Harvey

Mark A. Haskell

Joseph Henry

Irene Jillson

Marvin W. Kahn

Linda Lejero

Ann O'Keefe

Lynn E. Passy

Arthur Pearl

William J. Riley

Stanley S. Robin

A. M. Schneidmuhl

Joseph E. Scott

Jeanne K. Wagenfeld

Morton O. Wagenfeld

## DEDICATION

This book is dedicated to our parents: Margaret Robin and the memory of Joseph Robin, Izadore and Tillie Wagenfeld.

# Contents

# *Acknowledgements*

This book, like many other large efforts, reflects the help of a number of persons who work behind the scenes and are, thus, easily left unacknowledged. We hope that this section is a small step in making public our debt.

Dr. Bernard Bloom, the Series Editor, invited us to prepare this volume. He was an unfailingly helpful, supportive, and responsive colleague as well as gentle critic. For all these reasons, we thank him.

The staff of the Department of Sociology and the Center for Sociological Research has been helpful in a variety of typing, duplicating, and administrative tasks. We are grateful for their support. We would particularly like to thank Penne Ferguson who, in addition to typing innumerable drafts of the papers, coordinated many of the editorial details of the manuscript and spent long hours on the phone and in the library tracking down elusive references. How she was able to retain her sense of humor throughout all this is beyond us, but we are grateful.

Finally, and this is not an inconsiderable debt, we thank our colleagues who have contributed chapters to this volume. They have worked hard, often under unreasonably short deadlines, to produce papers that we believe are fresh, thoughtful and, we hope, original and provocative views of paraprofessionals.

S.S.R.
M.O.W.

Kalamazoo, Michigan
February, 1979

# *Introduction*

As detailed in this volume, paraprofessionals are employed in a wide variety of human services fields. The fact that they are established and so widely distributed has not spelled an end to the controversy about their employment and the effects of their employment. Assertions about the desirability and status of the paraprofessions abound. These assertions are made on the basis on anecdotal experience; evaluation research of varying stringency; promise of future benefits; ideological commitment; social analysis, and values realized and values thwarted.

Paraprofessionalism, outlasting the social-political context that advanced the idea, is depicted as an idea well-conceived, successfully applied, and flourishing. It has been mourned as a concept, promising and bright, that was stunted by flawed or inadequate execution. It is portrayed as a concept with confused and conflicting bases and aims doomed to failure by its internal inconsistencies. It has been condemned as a cruel hoax creating promises not attainable and the illusion of social change without substance.

These positions and assertions are presented and explored in this volume. Specific application of paraprofessionals to the various human services is also presented the participation of paraprofessionals in a variety of human services fields imposes an obligation to look carefully and with flexible criteria when evaluating their contribution. Consequently, the paraprofessional program that has met with partial success in one area may fail in another and succeed brilliantly in a third. The programmatic use of paraprofessionals may take radically different forms in the treatment of alcoholism and in education. Some values underlying paraprofessionalism may be realized in the Home Care Program, but others in the mental health field. It is because paraprofessionals must be understood in different ways in different fields, as well as in overview, that this volume is organized as it is.

The first section of the book. "Issues in Paraprofessionalism," presents an historical and theoretical overview. Arthur Pearl, one of the leading figures in this area, provides an historical perspective and an exploration of the rationale for the movement. He concludes with an analysis of the forces that may decide the fate of paraprofessionalism. Alan Gartner shows the current and projected needs for the services of paraprofessionals. He uses the mental health field to exemplify the variety of uses to which they are put. Finally, he prescribes a series of actions that need to be taken if the paraprofessionals are to be used to their fullest potential in the future.

Mark Haskell, economist, raises issues regarding the assessment of the paraprofessional movement in economic terms. He examines the manner in which evaluation techniques are created and applied to the use of paraprofessionals. Moreover, he points out that their evaluation and, ultimately their survival, may depend upon the use of both micro and macroeconomic approaches in assessment.

As the final selection in this section, we present Franklyn Arnhoff's article "New Careers: Where Have All the Flowers Gone." Arnhoff, in contrast to the two pieces at the beginning of the section, takes a negative view of the movement and its future. He develops the thesis that the use of paraprofessionals is waning and argues that the attempts to implement the basic tenets of paraprofessionalism were "cosmetic." He conclues that, in reality, para-professionalism has never been tried.

In the second section, "Paraprofessionals: The State of the Art," we present a series of articles that are analyses of the use and success of paraprofessionals in various human service fields. Alan Gartner details the wide-spread use of paraprofessionals in mental health. He concludes that their role has been a vital one and sees a strong place for them in the future.

Paraprofessionals in health-care delivery are discussed by Betty J. Cleckley. She presents the history and use of paraprofessionals in health care, but concludes, by citing a series of obstacles and difficulties in this field, that she sees growing more acute in the future.

Jeanne Wagenfeld assesses the use of the paraprofes-sional in education. She records a partial success and focuses upon a series of unresolved problems in para-professional integration into the U.S. educational system.

Paraprofesionals in criminal justice is offered by Jo-seph E. Scott who presents data bearing upon the extent of their use in the United States. He considers evalua-tions of their effectiveness and concludes with a favorable assessment.

The use of the paraprofessional in alcoholism counsel-ing is provided by A. M. Schneidmuhl, Gloria Doran, and Irene Jillson. They analyze the nature of the work of alcoholism counselors, their characteristics, and their current status in the field.

In the third section, "Paraprofessionals: Training, Re-search and Evaluation," we approach the "nuts and bolts" of paraprofessionalism. Judith Blanton and Sam Alley discuss the nature and the uses of evaluation in paraprofessional programs, detailing the special proce-dures and literature in this field.

William Riley, Morton O. Wagenfeld, and Stanley S. Robin present a study of paraprofessionals in community mental health centers. They conclude that professionals do not produce some of the changes in the centers predicted in the literature, but that the paraprofessionals themselves may be changed to reflect the attitudes of the medical professional. Allana Elovson presents the program of Home Start, in which paraprofessionals are the major workers. The training, functions, evaluations, problems and successes of these paraprofessionals are discussed.

Marvin W. Kahn, Joseph Henry and Linda Lejero detail the creation of indigenous mental health paraprofessionals in a program for the Papago Indians. They show the use of indigenous paraprofessionals to cope with inter-cultural problems of providing mental health services. Moreover, they explore the rationale, procedures and organization needed to use paraprofessionals in this fashion.

Mary R. Harvey and Lynn E. Passy write about the development of paraprofessionals in a university-based new careers program, discussing ways in which paraprofessionals can and are being trained within universities. They provide an analysis of the academic and political realities of this process.

In the fourth section, the editors provide a summary analysis of paraprofessionals in human services. In this chapter, an attempt is made to reconcile, integrate and rationalize the diverse perspectives presented in this volume. Wagenfeld and Robin then turn to questions of policy and develop some prescriptions for the development and use of paraprofessionals in the future.

The interest in paraprofessionalism is alive and vital for those in the academic fields, psychology, sociology, social work, as well as for those in more applied endeavors out in the field. Of concern to us are two basic premises that appear to be inherent in the development of the paraprofessional movement. First, the use of paraprofessionals would provide a means for large numbers of persons to improve the quality of their lives and to move out of poverty. In addition, by employing those who were former recipients, the human services would be humanized. These are values and concerns that join the applied and academic perspectives on paraprofessionals. The examination of paraprofessionalism and its honest evaluation, must continue as social circumstances and needs change.

S.S.R.
M.O.W

# I. ISSUES IN PARAPROFESSIONALISM

# The Paraprofessional in Human Service

Arthur Pearl,
*Committee of Education,
University of California, Santa Cruz*

"It is better to know nothing than to know what ain't so."—Josh Billings

Paraprofessionals have, depending on interpretation, either a very long or short history. The term itself is new, coined in the 1960s when a variety of human service programs recruited indigenous poor into service delivery. The effort was part of the grandly announced "war on poverty." That war, in large measure, recapitulated the tragedy of the *other* war in Viet Nam. There were differences in those wars to be sure, but in the phrase that

23

typifies the 70's—the bottom line—those wars were identical. We lost both. And the indigenous poor were both wars' greatest casualties.

The term paraprofessional itself reflects the confusion that has deprived us of vision and mission. Not knowing what else to call them they became paraprofessionals. It was a consummation no one wished. No proud mother gushed over "my son the paraprofessional." No child dreamed of the day that she/he would grow up to be a paraprofessional. Paraprofessional was and is, an unsatisfactory compromise. The term is not a synthesis of warring forces—the conflicts and contradictions remain unresolved. The traditionalist perceives the new hirelings to be no different than the other menials who play insignificant supportive roles to the professional in human services; hence, to them, paraprofessionals are nonprofessionals at best, unprofessional at worst. The romantics riding what they believed (some still do) the tide of revolution proclaimed the indigenous poor to be the new professionals. Many believed that need was for a fundamental change in the *nature* of service involved a developmental process of preparation interspersed with field experiences: a "praxis" of action and reflection as advocated by Paulo Friere, pushed for preprofessional (Friere, 1970). Paraprofessional was a term that had no adherents; it just raised fewer hackles than anything else proposed. Like everything else in situations of detente, it was the least unsatisfactory alternative.

The term is as ambiguous as everything else in the history of the paraprofessional. Para is a prefix that has many meanings. Para can be beside as in parallel, or a derivative as in paraldehyde, or abnormal as in paranoia, or even that which protects from, as in parasol. Paraprofessionals have met all and none of these definitions. They have been seen as alternatives to, derivatives from, distortions of, and very rarely protectors from—the professional. What they are depends upon one's view of human services. For those who believe that professionals provide uniformly high quality services the paraprofessional is an assistant or a distraction. Those who believe with George Bernard Shaw that "all professions are conspiracies against the laity" look to the paraprofessional for reformation or revolution. That is the backdrop against which an historical perspective must be drawn.

This represents the dilemma of our age, but history preceeds 1964 and at an earlier time when life was less complex, and revisionist historians the exception not the rule, those who now serve as paraprofessionals were assistants or apprentices. In the former instance, they could not expect to rise in station in the latter position they could. History is spotted with eras and situations where the less than the professional played vital roles in human service delivery.

At the end of the 19th century, Joseph Lancaster and Andrew Bell initiated a plan whereby schools with 300 or more students could be taught by a single teacher assisted by numerous monitors. The school operated on a principle of individualized tutoring in which older students assisted younger. It has a modern ring to it and recently has been rediscovered. In both England and in the United States the Lancaster concept rapidly gained popularity. In New York, the program was sponsored by Governor DeWitt Clinton. In its heyday, it is estimated that as many as 30,000 students attended Lancaster schools. By 1830, it was on the wane and Lancaster schools disappeared never to return in 1853. Viewed from a distance, Lancaster took on different nuances. Martin Mayer (1961) in his essay, *The Schools,* blasts Lancasterianism:

> The efficiency of the operation was extremely low, and the waste of children's good time was unforgivable. Something of this sort is probably necessary when a highly-populated area first tries to produce a literate community. The monitorial system bears more than a slight resemblance to the "each one teach one" program which is bringing the benefits of

reading and writing to the peasant of Asia. But it is
not a system anyone would voluntarily choose for his
own children. (p. 41)

Bassett (1978), however, sees Lancaster with very different colored glasses:

Since the teacher had to do a copious amount of
creative planning to keep the system working, the
monitorial school demonstrated a need for teacher
training, for professionally-prepared materials, for
use of teaching techniques and aids in the learning
process, and for the efficient organization of instruction. The value of having one pupil help another for
the benefit of both ("to teach is to learn" said Joub-
ert) was brought to light. It has be rediscovered in
recent years. (p.107)

Both Bassett and Mayer agree that parents foresook
Lancaster for professional teachers school—Mayer on the
grounds that Lancaster was inferior, Bassett because the
system had been thus stigmatized, "Parents wanted their
children to have a 'proper' education, delivered directly
to them by a 'proper' teacher" (Bassett, 1978). The question whether paraprofessionals are "proper" remains
with us. Although discredited and cast into history's junk
heap, Lancasterian schools were never proved to be less
effective than the schools that replaced them. One lesson
to learn from history of paraprofessionals —it is not what
they have done or didn't do that determined their success,
it is how established power chose to treat them on issues
extraneous to effectiveness on the job.
  Lancaster schools were privately run, they were swept
aside with the development of large scale public support
of education and that in turn gave rise to professional
teachers. This, without supportive data, was supposed to
have raised standards and established criteria that for-
bade the extensive use of nonprofessionals. Another les-

son of history—nonprofessionals are employed only when professionals aren't available to do the job.

Jump ahead a hundred years to another waystation in the history of the paraprofessional. The year 1953, the place, Bay City, Michigan, the paraprofessional, the teacher aide. In this program, teacher aides were paired with teachers in elementary school classrooms with 45 or more students. The goal of the program was to enhance teacher efficiency by using aides to perform menial tasks that otherwise would be the responsibility of highly-trained professionals. The aides were professionally oriented persons who participated in preservice training in specific skills and a general orientation in child development. The criteria used to evaluate the Bay City teachers aide program were, 1) student performance on standardized tests; 2) parent opinions; 3) teacher assessments; 4) pupil evaluations; 5) aide records of activities and; 6) controlled observations of teachers and aides. The results were favorable but inconclusive—there was no difference in student learning but parents and teachers had positive attitudes toward the project, teachers claimed to have more time to teach and the observations revealed that teachers spent less time correcting papers, disciplining students, taking roll and more time in lesson preparation. The fear and persistent criticism of Bay City was the lesser trained persons were replacing the qualified teachers (Park, et al., 1956).

One learned from the Bay City experiment a refinement of a previously-taught lesson; paraprofessionals not only are employed only when professionals aren't available to do the job but when they appear capable of replacing professionals become threats—"rate busters," "scabs," and the like.

Now rip off the pages of our calendar at a furious pace and jump to the mid 1960s' and the war on poverty. Without regard to the lessons of history, enter the era of paraprofessionalism. It has been a short and bitter era. For the next half decade, millions of people were hired, some poor, to serve as teacher aides in pre-school, elementary, and secondary school programs, homemaker aides, assistants to lawyers, or community mental health workers in make-shift street front clinics or as community workers for police departments. Some worked in variously defined duties in housing projects, in a variety of youth service projects or in public health departments. Some became aides for probation and parole. If you could name and place it, you could have yourself a paraprofessional.

The paraprofessional was hired without a unifying theory and, in many instances, without clear notions of responsibilities. They were hired in a poverty program that Daniel Patrick Moynihan argued did not have work for male adults as one of its objectives. They were hired to help overcome the "deficits that caused poor people to remain poor."

To understand the history of the paraprofessional it is imperative that the sense of the time be recaptured. We had discovered the existence of poverty in our affluent society. The poor were, as Michael Harrington (who more than any other person drew attention to their presence in his book, *The Other America* put it, "invisible" (Harrington, 1962). It was a strange period. Magic was in the air. We had a handsome president. He attracted youthful idealists, mostly from Harvard, who were full of ideas and empty of experience to help him forge a "new frontier." It was the best of times. We were advancing on all fronts. It was, as Henry Luce had decreed it to be, "The American Century." We had only a few advisors in Vietnam. Between 1960 and 1965, the number of unemployed had been reduced by 500,000. Despite declining unemployment, the consumer price index increased less than 2% per year in the same period. If people weren't making it in the United States, something had to be wrong with *them*. The theme that dominated the war on poverty, at least in its earliest years, was "accumulated environmental deficit" and that in turn established the use to which paraprofessionals would be put. "Accumulated environmental" deficit explained poverty as a stochastic process. For want of cognitive stimulation in the earliest formulative years, children of poverty entered school with deficiencies in language and analytical ability. Unable to effectively compete with children from favored backgrounds, this in turn led to early termination of schooling which caused "structural" unemployment, and which was an inability to enter those sectors of the job market that required advanced degree education. Those were the jobs that not only paid the most, they were most prestigious, most permanent, but also (at that time) were becoming the most numerous.

To overcome their accumulated environmental deficits, the poor required compensatory treatments. The most celebrated of these was Operation Head Start, which began as a summer program and was extended first, to year 'round programs, and later to three year programs with the addition of Operation Follow Through. Other programs with compensatory orientation were the Elementary and Secondary Education Act, Manpower Development and Training Act, Upward Bound and the juvenile delinquency projects, (e.g., New York's Mobilization for Youth and Haryou). Other programs in housing or welfare or employment that were not designed to repair the poor operated with deficiencies of the poor in mind. And all of these agencies created jobs for people whose duty it was to provide service for the deficited poor. According to the official rhetoric of the juvenile delinquency programs, the desired result would be access to the legitimate "opportunity structure" for the delinquent. The same logic applied to other populations to be served.[1] Whatever its intent, the primary beneficiaries of

[1]See Richard A. Cloward and Lloyd E. Ohlin. *Delinquency and Opportunity*, New York, Free Press, 1960, which did much to inspire not only the delinquency program but also the Community Action titles of the poverty program. Access to opportunity would come through organizing for political "clout" not by job creation. At that time, there was a growing belief that jobs were fast becoming obsolete

the poverty program were the persons hired to provide the service, many of whom were established professionals, others who were persons without the prerequisite degrees but with substantial progress in that direction. In the beginning stages, very few persons who were hired to provide direct service to the poor were themselves poor. The author likes to think it was I who coined the phrase that the President's Committee on Juvenile Delinquency and the Office of Economic Opportunity "were opening up the opportunity structures for the middle class."

It could not be otherwise, considering the theoretical orientations of the program and the understanding of poverty. People with accumulated environmental deficits could not be expected to help others similarly affected. They needed to be first brought up to a specified level of functioning and then it would be possible for them to offer assistance to others. Anything else would be an erosion of standards and would be a disservice to the poor people whose problems largely stem from a history of disservice —at least that's the gist of the argument.

A few of us weren't convinced. In spring, 1963 under the auspices of the New York State Division of Youth and the National Institute of Mental History, Frank Riessman and I brought together a panel of experts on poverty and although the dominant view expressed was that poverty was the result of personal inadequacies or *past* injustices, a few of us took the tack that poverty resulted from locking people out of what was rapidly becoming a credential society rather than from any possible impediment in character or personality. We drew from scattered experiences that showed that poor people, if given opportunity to perform, could do many things that "experts" had concluded were beyond their capabilities. I was particularly impressed by the activities of another past paraprofessional program, "the medics," of the United States

---

and would be replaced by automated activities. Thus, it follows that political access to the machine generating goods and service would obliterate poverty.

Army. Here in a very short period of time, prompted by the wartime demands for medical service and the scarcity of qualified professionals to provide that service, high quality medical care was created by using people, often from backgrounds of poverty, with no previous experience, training or skills in the practice of medicine. There was also the experiences of persons in therapeutic communities who were better able to manage their lives in prisons and mental hospitals when they took over responsibilities rather than being "served" by others (Jones, 1953). There were the Bay City Teacher Aides. There were the 1930 "gang" studies of the Chicago YMCA where erstwhile gangleaders took on constructive roles. There was the potentialities of youth leadership that was demonstrated in Highfields type programs for minimally delinquent youth (McCorkle, Elias and Bixby, 1958).

From this exchange came first, *Mental Health of the Poor,* a book of readings edited by Riessman, Cohen, and Pearl (1964) that questioned the validity of "professional" treatment of low income persons and minorities who suffer from emotional distress. Following shortly after, was the logical sequel, *New Careers for the Poor,* authored primarily by Riessman and Pearl (1965) which presented a general theory that could be used to solve uniquely and simultaneously the troublesome problems of poverty racism (and other injustices) as well as inadequate services through recruitment of low income people into the fastest growing professional occupations. *New Careers* specifically rejected "deficit theories" of poverty and offered, instead, the thesis that poverty resulted from a lack of options—the exclusion from the most lucrative legitimate means of earning a living. To better understand how such a theory could solve poverty, racism, *and* inadequate service, it is necessary to review its basic features.

New Careers operates with the premise that a good society organizes its work to meet the characteristics of its people instead of trying to shape its people to meet the dictates of capriciously-defined work. This latter approach reinforces prejudice and bias because persons are denied an opportunity to show what they can do on the job since they do not have the *prerequisites* for the job.

It proposes that work and education be integrated, that the student is able to put to immediate use the knowledge obtained in schooling situations instead of the present situation which requires the student to remain useless for as many as two decades in school. It is impossible in this latter system for the student to validate the learning. The student is forced to take the word of some adult authority. This is never a totally satisfactory arrangement and in times like these where all authority is suspect, it is particularly unworkable. If the adult authority is wrong or obsolete, the student is provided inappropriate concepts and skills that in turn leads to inappropriate and inadequate service.

But for New Careers really to be operative, it must be a force that goes beyond merely rearranging existing work. It also has to be a force to create work. There can be New Careers only when there are as many opportunities to work as there are persons available to work. New Careers requires full employment and vice versa. Only with true full employment can there be a solution to poverty. Only if one identifies unmet social needs, organize work to overcome these needs and allow anyone regardless of background and experience to try his/her hand at that work, will it be possible for race or other prejudices to be overcome. New Careers runs counter to the idea that work is becoming obsolete and that, as a society, we should be encouraging our citizens to aspire to leisure and leave work to the machines and the few technicians that will be needed to run those machines (Theobald, 1964).

New Careers also opposes the classical economic theory that human needs and desires would, somehow create work through the mysterious and "invisible hand of the market." The market theory has many obstacles. Two are apparent and devastating. One, those things most needed by people simply are not profitable (e.g., housing, medical and leisure pursuits) for those with low or no income; and second, professionals have effectively conspired against allowing people to work where there is opportunity. Only established doctors allow persons who have graduated from institutions approved by them, to engage in the practice of medicine. Thus, while there is clearly identified needs for medical service there is no opportunity for "the market" to satisfy that need.

New Careers, thus presented an alternative to the guaranteed-annual-wage Dr. Panglosses who insisted that, while we did not live "in the best of all possible worlds," we were fast getting there and to those fundamentalists who argued that we needed to retrace our steps and go back to where we started from.

The career in New Careers is important. Most of those who have supported programs to create work as a means to overcome poverty, as far back as the great depression of the 1930s and as recently as today, think in terms of jobs that are temporary, expecting that permanent work will come about through stimulation of the total economy. New Careers rejects "jobs." Jobs do not offer the promise eliminating racism or poverty, and jobs are unlikely to improve service. Since "jobs" are short-term, they offer no economic security. Moreover, since "jobs" cannot really provide quality services. There is a tendency to sneer at those who are working in them and this adds to, rather than detracts from, race, class, and sex bias. Careers are permanent and openended. The needs that are addressed by careers are expected to continue into the future. If there should come a time when there appears to be less needed work than there are workers, then the issue first should be resolved by altering hours of work, not by reducing the number of people who work. Although given the condition of cities, health problems, the deterioration of the environment, lack of housing, transportation, sad state of education, the need for places and services in leisure, the time when we could conceivably run out of needed work is far away, if, indeed, it is even remotely possible. New Careers, therefore, proposes that entry positions be made available for anyone. Once such a position is established, persons receive training and education to learn on the job; those with ability and drive can achieve the next step and in a similar fashion be able to negotiate all steps to the attainment of the ultimate professional position. For those unwilling or unable to advance, each rung in the ladder could be a career position.

That was New Careers as it was formulated in 1965. Operating with slogans, "service from rather than service to," and "taxpayers rather than tax eaters," it became a part of the poverty program as the Scheuer Amendment to the Economic Opportunity Act. It was also introduced in various other governmental-sponsored human services. It was never a major thrust. It was a hedge against the primary effort that continued to be compensatory in nature. But it was the beginning of new thinking and despite the lack of enthusiasm with which it was treated, the failure to come close to meeting its intent, and often confronted by outright sabotage, it remains today as the only viable alternative to either a guaranteed annual income (which is fast disappearing as a defensible ideal) or the continuation of inequality and impoverishment.

## New Careers in Theory and in Practice

New Careers was launched with virtually no preparation. It was transplanted to cities where no one had the slightest notion of its meaning, and it went where it had few, if any, advocates. If ever a program was designed to fail, it was New Careers. It didn't. It survived although it really never was tried in anything near its intended form. In many cities, New Careers was but a slight modification of the deficit oriented manpower training programs it was designed to replace. It is difficult to state with any degree of accuracy what actually happened in most New Careers programs. There were hundreds of programs that advertised themselves to be New Careers or Career Opportunity Programs (which was the term used in the Educational Professional Development Act). They had little in common with each other, but it is possible to make some defensible generalizations.

Almost all New Career programs did put to work persons who had been deemed to be unemployable.

Almost all New Career programs generated a career ladder, although most were extremely truncated.

Almost all New Career programs gave release time for workers to receive training and education.

Many New Career programs provided college credits for training and education.

Many New Career programs were able to work arrangements with institutions of higher education to provide credit for verified job related learning (although more frequently college credit was given without identifying the competencies that were learned).

Many New Careerists were able to use the program to escape poverty and establish themselves firmly as successful professionals. New Careerists have gone on to serve as high ranking administrators in HEW and in the National Institute of Mental Health.

Few New Career programs established clearly defined procedures whereby persons could advance *in the program* to the highest ranked professional status.

*No* New Career program was able to produce a fundamental change in professional preparation.[2] Professional schools remained intransigent and refused either to change their programs or to engage in the kind of conscientious evaluation to determine if change was needed.

[2]The University of Oregon built a New Careers orientation into the fabric of its School of Community Service and Public Affairs. Its accomplishments are reported in another chapter.

If anything, there has been a retreat to the more traditional approaches of professional preparation.

New Careers, from its beginning, has been an appendage to the anti-poverty, anti-discrimination movements and thus, it has no noticeable effect on either the magnitude of poverty or the state of justice in the United States. Benefits to individuals in these areas, however, are undeniable.

On balance, despite its gaps and inadequate execution, New Careers worked. People with unstable work history tended to become vocationally stable. They were competent and efficient. When they reached a professional status, they favorably compared with persons who gained their status traditionally.[3]

Two programs, because they were done under "glass" and thus its accomplishments and its problems were visible to all, deserve brief but special mention. This was the Community Apprentice Program at Harvard and the California Offender New Career Project. In the Harvard Project, 10 young people between the ages of 16 and 21 with deplorable school records, work histories, and involvements with the law were offered a two-week orientation which preceded work appointments as researchers, child care attendants, and group workers in an inner city "settlement house." For the next four months, they worked half a day and received training during the other half. They received minimum wages for this period of time and were paid only while they worked, receiving no renumeration for the training. Amazingly, despite their records, all 10 remained with the project for its 18-month duration. They demonstrated an ability to learn beyond any previously expressed expectations. Moreover, they

[3]See, for example, Wilson, et al., *National Institute for New Careers,* University Research Corp., Washington, D.C., 1969; Hoff, et al., Home Aide Pilot Training Project: Final Evaluation Report. Alameda County Health Department, Oakland, Calif., 1968; Costa, C., *A Comparative Study of Career Opportunities Program Graduates as First Year Teachers,* New York, New Careers Training Lab, Queens College, 1975.

remained free of legal entanglements. Where once they had been sources of problems for the community, they became constructive citizens. The program never ran smoothly; there were constant emergencies and crises but nothing that erupted into a calamity. The change was so spectacular that persons who did not know the youth at the beginning could not believe their social history (Pearl and Riessman, 1965; Sherif and Sherif, 1965; and Fishman, 1965).

In the California Offender Project (Grant and Grant, 1967), persons with long-term criminal histories and a parole prediction index that indicated a very high probability of return to prison within two years, were recruited into an experimental program. The subjects in this experiment were screened on the basis of personality and intelligence but were nonetheless extremely "high risks" to return to a life of crime. For a period of 2 to 6 months prior to release into the community, this group of new convicts were brought to the prison at Vacaville to engage in an intensive training program that emphasized communication skills, program development and research. The results were spectacular. Of 18 members of this group only one returned to prison in the two years of the study. Although there have been a few relapses since the end of this project in 1967, there also has been continued progress for most of the persons involved. Two went on to earn Ph.Ds, several have Master's Degrees, and at this writing, two are high-ranking governmental officials (Grant and Grant, 1967).

New Careers was successful but there are virtually no New Careers programs left; little has changed in the institutions that were supposed to be changed by a New Career approach. Why? What lessons can we learn from *that* history (Grant and Grant, 1975)?[4]

----

[4]It might be a better presumption to insist that New Careers succeeded since it is so difficult to fully evaluate so complex an intervention.

## Nothing Fails Like Success

Success is meaningless if the game has been changed. It makes no difference how good a Mahjong player you are if no one plays Mahjong anymore, and that is what happened to New Careers and other paraprofessional programs. During the 1960s, the primary social thrust was responding to a civil rights movement that captured the imagination of a wide segment of the population. This was followed by the war on poverty. Those movements can and were superseded by movements against the Vietnam war and lastly, by a war against ecological damage to the environment. The movements were short term and largely spontaneous. They were more rhetorical than substantive and ultimately, the rhetoric cancelled out the substance. The underlying logic of the wars against poverty and injustice was based on an infinite earth thesis— we could cure our social ills by outgrowing them. The increasing productivity of an ever more efficient technological society would produce such a plethora of goods and services so that soon no one need be poor anymore; the economic factors that reinforced discrimination and bias were fast disappearing. The civil rights and anti-poverty movements were primarily moral. They stemmed from a conclusion that the problems we had were a matter of will, not capacity. The "ecology" movement was also moral but it ran completely counter to the actions that preceded it. Its basic tenets were that not only was the world finite, but its growth was exceeding its capacity to maintain itself. The ecologists deflected concern away from the plight of humans to other species. There was more concern expressed for three-toed salamanders and baby harp seals than there was for ghetto or barrio residents. It was a hectic period but it left people with little to build upon, and its basic legacy was exhaustion. It was, however, a decade characterized by social concern, even if that concern was romantic and superficial. We find ourselves in a totally different situation today. If the mood of the 60s was other and altruistically directed, the 70s have been a decade dominated by selfishness. Every aspect of life has taken on a preoccupation with self to the decline in concern about others. There was seeds of this turnabout in public sentiment in the 1960s "self liberation" movements; it has come to dominate all of popular psychology and the arts. Consequently, it has had three devastating manifestations for the paraprofessional:

1.  We don't need them—we can take care of ourselves.
2.  We can't afford them—inflation and taxes make them exorbitant.
3.  They don't give us what we need.

## WE DON'T NEED THEM—WE CAN TAKE CARE OF OURSELVES

Paraprofessionals function in bureaucratic structures. They are effectively precluded by law and licensing to go out on their own. Very rarely can a paraprofessional hang out a shingle and offer educational, medical, legal, or police services, etc. Thus he/she is dependent upon a "system" for employment. If the sentiment of people becomes anti-system, if the political right and left direct these energies against system, if the right believes "systems are socialistic," and left, "fascist," then the paraprofessional loses support because of a lack of constituency. The 1970s if they are anything, are anti-system.

There is widespread distrust of government and big business. In a sense, we have never gotten over Vietnam and, since Watergate followed shortly after, and Koreagate became the Republicans' desperate attempt to get even, the credibility of big government and business diminished. This effort was particularly effective when it was directed against those programs that were supposed to help the poor. Cuts in poverty and other human services programs were justified on the grounds that they were "rip-offs" and "frauds." The attack was general and, during Richard Nixon's stay in the White House, programs that succeeded were lumped with those that failed. The net effect was the impression that the approach itself was hopeless.

In such situations, it is not surprising that people turn away from government. Since, there was a companion theme operating at the same time—"self-help"—rejection of the government didn't appear to have any negative consequence. Self-help comes in every possible guise and was used on every possible ailment. Gurus and evangelists cropped up everywhere. Every list of the 10 best selling books had at least one that presented self cures for everything from cancer to unpopularity. Cults not only mushroomed, they centrifugalized. The splintering destroyed any possibility for *political* responses to wrongdoing. Thus despite complaint and withdrawal of energy, government continues to grow, because people are so wrapped up in finding their true selves and proclaiming that whatever they are is OK, they can't bring themselves to do anything about it. What the preoccupation with self means for the paraprofessional is simply this: There is declining support for their services among the affluent who are now in the business of helping themselves, and the poor, who desperately need help, are forced into self help because those in a position to underwrite such services are too pre-occupied with themselves.

The sad part of all of that is that despite TA, TM, EST, Eckencar, bioenergetics, bipolarity, etc., venereal disease, alcoholism, crime increases, cities become more unlivable, school violence and vandalism increases, emotional problems increase, drug abuse continues, and young children increasingly get battered. These are problems that require something more than self-help and yet, there is no organized and sustained response to them.

Therein probably lies the most severe energy crisis of our time.

## WE CAN'T AFFORD THEM—INFLATION AND TAXES MAKE THEM EXORBITANT

While a group of people preoccupy themselves and strip their inhibitions with explicit and titilating art forms and social experiementation, the world goes on and is directed by inertia and established interest groups. These two forces, if not checked, increase the likelihood of war, poverty, racism, and sexism (and other injustices), and even more dehumanizing social organizations. They have produced the heretofore impossible simultaneous high inflation and high unemployment. These two undesirable economic conditions are supposed to, according to traditional wisdom, work at cross purposes. Inflation is supposed to bring down unemployment whereas deflation is supposed to create joblessness. Conversely, joblessness supposedly causes deflation and full employment supposedly causes inflation. That this economic law isn't working has profound implications for paraprofessionals.

Normally, high unemployment is a crisis for a government. Thus, it moves to decrease it. Since the 1929 depression, governments that function in societies that call themselves capitalist, try to stem the tide of rising unemployment by stimulating the economy. One of the means used to do that is public service employment. A consequence of public service employment is the hiring of paraprofessionals. Thus, one has found periods of high unemployment, jobs created in schools, health centers, welfare offices, recreation agencies, housing departments, etc. More recently, paraprofessionals have been involved in ecological projects. But this is not the response in periods of inflation. During inflation, the economy is "cooled." One means to do that is to *reduce* the number of persons employed by the government. If inflation is seen as the *most* serious economic problem, then political support for employment (which is another way of saying paraprofessionalism) declines.

This is precisely what happened in the double digit inflation crisis that began in 1974 and has remained a cause of concern since. President Ford laid it out succinctly. To him it was quite simple, "Umemployment hurts a minority of us, inflation hurts everybody." And the best way to reduce inflation was to refuse to support government employment-creating programs. He carried that logic one step further. He would rather increase unemployment benefits than increase government job creation. His reasoning was that the government employment tends to remain, building with it a support system, and a difficult to dismantle bureaucracy, whereas unemployment insurance will disappear when the economy picks up.

His opponent for the presidency in 1976 did not take issue with this type of analysis. To the contrary, Jimmy Carter ran primarily on the theme that he could bring both morality and efficiency to government. It is not surprising then, that he, too, after barely a year in office, declared "inflation" to be the nation's number one problem. That of course means support for paraprofessional employment would be markedly reduced, if not completely curtailed.

In education, where perhaps most paraprofessionals have been employed, the crunch is already being experienced. Declining enrollments, increased paraprofessional association power and an unwillingness of taxpayers to produce dollars has resulted in layoffs of teacher aides and other paraprofessionals.

This is somewhat different in medicine, but whether this trend will continue is not at all certain. The number of persons employed as health service workers and health technicians (other than M.D.s, Registered Nurses, and Dieticians) did increase by nearly 300,100 between 1972 and 1975 (*1977 Statistical Abstract,* p. 77). Lower rung paraprofessionals' positions, however, are not solid. The wars between paraprofessional groups are intense (psychiatric technicians vs. nurses vs. community workers), and physicians, if anything, have increased their control over health delivery systems. If effective patient resistance against the skyrocketing costs of health care arises, with change in the political situation, the inevitable result will be losses in paraprofessional employment.

All of these machinations come against a backdrop of "taxpayer revolts." Taxpayers' complaints are solidly founded on fact. Taxes *are* eroding income. In 1955, property and income taxes amounted to 19% of wages. In 1970, this had risen to 25%. The rise in sentiment for more conservatively fiscal policies can be seen in the modest decline that has occurred since 1970. In 1974, property and income tax dropped to 23% of wages (*1977 Statistical Abstract*, U.S. Department of Commerce). The problem with "the taxpayer revolt" approach to complex social problems is that a campaign is conducted at the lowest intellectual level, and appeal is to emotion and not to thought; there is no systematic analysis of governmental expenditures, unsubstantial wild changes appear credible, and exceptional cases become the rule. In such situations, any reduction in governmental expense take their primary toll on those persons with least prestige, seniority, and social support. Ergo—taxpayer revolts lead to decline in paraprofessional employment.

## THEY DON'T GIVE US WHAT WE NEED

Part of the decline in paraprofessionalism is retreat into selfishness. The selfishness takes many forms—insulation, greed, lack of concern—each of which has a negative influence on less than professional employment in the human services, particularly those services that are part of government. Selfishness cannot in itself explain diminished interest in "social programs." Part of the problem is in the nature of the service. Dissatisfaction with public services is one of the major reasons that government has lost credibility.

The schools stand out as an example of a once admired institution that has fallen from grace. For almost two decades, schools have been subjected to fearsome attacks from both left and right. The right have been concerned about the decline in basic skills, the loss of healthy work attitudes, and the high incidence of youth involvement in crime, drugs, and violence. The left attack the schools as oppressive institutions that rob children of their childhood, natural curiosity, and individuality. It is difficult to justify the employment of paraprofessionals in a system that has few defenders and cannot be defended on the basis of evidence. As education comes increasingly under attack, teachers, as a body, do not rise and present either logic or evidence for their performance; instead, they fall back on professionalism which consists of:

1. Withdrawal from debate with critics.
2. Puffery—the argot of mysterious and arcane phrases that are supposed to be scientific.
3. Reinforcement of all licensing and contractual systems to make them immune from general public influence.
4. Closure of ranks, and that translates into a one for all and all for one, which in turn means that there can be no serious internal evaluation of relevance or competence.
5. Virulent scapegoatery of generalized others, particularity parents, but also television, non-student trespassers, and organized criminals.
6. Arrogant dismissal of parent and student grievances.

Unaccountable systems generate little public support but these systems have the ability to deflect criticism to its most visible and most vulnerable hirelings. These, all too often, are the paraprofessionals. Even if the para-professional is not the scapegoat or the person set up to be spokesperson for the service, he/she can be made vulnerable by the inevitable response to the charge of inadequate service—"we will upgrade it." Upgrading means increasing professionalism. Thus, if children do not appear to be able to read, reading specialists are created, if children are unruly, specialists in social and emotional disorders are created, etc., all of this doesn't bode well for the paraprofessional.

History if it has any value, if it is to be more than the "bunk" that Henry Ford decided it was, or the "lies agreed to" which is attributed to Napoleon, must be a lesson for the future. Where *do* we go from here with paraprofessionals? Can we conceptualize a less chaotic involvement of persons without professional credentials working in the delivery of human services? Is it possible to reduce the professional—paraprofessional antagonisms? Can we generate a lasting political constituency for the paraprofessional? Is it possible to alter job descriptions and educational systems so that the steps from paraprofessional to professional are clearly defined and negotiable for all categories of paraprofessionals? Can we develop a system in which the paraprofessional is not a second class citizen—available to women, minorities and other disadvantaged persons while the top rung professional remains as a preserve for the economically advantaged male? Can we organize an economy that doesn't use the paraprofessional as ballast to throw out whenever the economy has to rise? And lastly, can we visualize service systems, in which paraprofessionals play vital roles, which are responsive to client needs, and can provide convincing evidence of quality? How we will answer these questions will determine whether we have learned anything from history. Four issues require some special treatment and are presented as a conclusion to this essay. These are:

1. The paraprofessional and the economy.
2. The paraprofessional and quality of service.
3. The paraprofessional and a political constituency.
4. The paraprofessional and institutions of higher learning.

## THE PARAPROFESSIONAL AND THE ECONOMY

It is impossible to plan coherently about the role of human service providers unless such planning is integrated within a total economic scheme. Anything short of a total plan guarantees the recaptualization of previous history where the paraprofessional is treated as an economic yo-yo to be used sparingly in normal times, to be greatly relied upon in times of emergency (such as a war), to be a device that reduces abnormally high unemployment, and to be sacrificed as an appeasement to the gods that cause inflation.

New career strategy was predicated on full employment. Full employment is vital to the stablization of any type of paraprofessional employment. Those who desire the employment of any category of workers must also work for the employment of all persons who desire work. The failure to incorporate paraprofessionalism into a macroeconomic understanding contributed significantly to the fall of the paraprofessional in the past decade. Full employment is not an easily achieved goal. A technical society appears to work at cross purposes to employment. As the major industries increase sales, they intensify capital holdings and use these monies to increase efficiency which means the number of persons employed declines both relatively and absolutely. Between 1960 and 1977, the 500 largest industrial corporations increased their sales more than five-fold with less than twice the number of workers. Between 1973 and 1977, these firms increased their sales by $420 billion and employed

200,000 fewer people (*Fortune Magazine,* 1961, 1974, and 1978).

Economic planning that looks to the "private sector" for producing work not only is going to tolerate high levels of unemployment but will produce other undersirable conditions as well. One of these is increased probability of energy crises. Efficient industries reduce employment as machines replace workers, by increasing fuel consumption. This trade-off has led to a situation where more and more U.S. energy is imported. This has profound implications for world peace. Developed nations look to the undeveloped nations for oil and unreplenishable minerals. This imbalancing, in effect, requires undeveloped nations to remain undeveloped—otherwise they too would be making demands on an already severely limited resource and thereby threaten supply for the developed nations. The widening gulf between the developed and undeveloped nation is readily observable in the United Nations but also in specific hot spots in Africa, Latin America, and Asia.

We have two courses of action to avoid catastrophy of either a world war and/or an economic collapse—we can generate new energy or we can use less. Efforts to generate new energy—nuclear, solar, geothermal, methane (from waste), etc.—have not been proven to be efficient or safe. History informs us there are always unanticipated negative consequences in energy exchanges, that is one of the manifestations of the second law of thermodynamics.

One way to use less energy is to move from a "goods" oriented economy to a human-service economy. A human service economy elevates the importance of interpersonal relationships. The heart of the economy elevates the importance of interpersonal relationships. The heart of the economy are those activities that people offer directly to other people. A human service economy features education, health services (which is not the same thing as medicine), environmental repair, support of leisure, esthetics, care for the aged and the young, protection of the vulnerable, and service to persons who currently are required to help themselves.

## The Paraprofessional and Quality of Service

A shift from a techno-industrial society to one that reduced the influence of such a force in our society would be difficult. Corporations have enormous power. The 500 largest industrial corporations not only do more than half the nation's business, but they have amassed more than $800 billion in assets. Moreover, they are solidly represented in all of the political structures of our society. They exercise considerable control over the media, interjecting ideological supports for the private enterprise system, advertising the quality and importance of their wares, and blacklisting or denegrating persons and ideas that they are "disloyal" to the "system" although today there is much less direct attack on dissidents. Now they are merely ignored or ridiculed. If the situation declines and we are plunged into a depression or war, the corporate influence is almost assuredly to be experienced more overtly and forcefully. The political pressures generated and sustained by corporate enterprise is not going to stand benignly and idly by and allow the economy to change from a goods oriented to a human service economy. The only way that can happen is for a sufficiently powerful, well-focused and organized counter political force to bring it about.

Politically overcoming entrenched interests of the magnitude that exist in the United States will be extraordinarily difficult; it is impossible unless a case can be made for the human services. Human services suffer from two kinds of crises of credibility—the nature of the service itself and the "bureaucracy."

No human services is immune from either of these difficulties, although the problems are most apparent in education and medicine. A change from a goods to a human service economy requires a dramatic shift in the way of life for a group of people. Change of that magnitude is threatening under the best of conditions, but if the new goal has already been tarnished, where does one get the energy to produce the shift? Neither education nor medicine can gain sufficient supporters unless new visions are formulated. These visions must excite. They must, in theory, show how they can provide universal government. Government will continue to license, to underwrite education, and otherwise prepare persons for professional and paraprofessional work, and will be involved in criminal and civil actions against work. Government will prosecute and protect persons accused of malpractice, incompetence, or disloyalty. The vision that describes a credible service must also describe and defend a credible government.

## THE PARAPROFESSIONAL AND A POLITICAL CONSTITUENCY

Visions can generate enthusiasm, visions can bring a splintered people together, but change requires a *sustained* political constituency and that is what the paraprofessional has never had. It has been expediency, not conscious political action, that has sparked the periodic uses of the paraprofessional. The paraprofessional has been created by those in high positions and imposed upon the people, who were to be served, often the efforts were more to pacify than to provide assistance. (And even if that wasn't the intention, that was the only possible result.) [5]

A vision cannot, by itself, cause change; a human service society that offers employment to everyone can only become a reality when people are organized to bring it

[5] For example, a job training program may not intend to provide an illusion of service. That is the only possible consequence if there are no jobs for the graduated trainee.

about. Such organization must be permanent, generate a dues paying membership, provide on a regular basis information to its members and interested others, and be actively involved in the political processes of the society.

One way to begin to build a constituency for the paraprofessional is to mobilize those persons who have been helped by the paraprofessional. If persons served by paraprofessionals are unwilling to rally behind that service then one needs no more evidence of its failure to satisfy.

Ultimately, the future paraprofessionals will be determined by their ability to provide a needed service. The paraprofessional cannot be defended merely because he/she is out of work and, therefore, some makeshift and unessential jobs must be hastily created. And yet, this latter approach has dominated the thinking regarding paraprofessionals in this last decade. It is no wonder that there are fewer, and fewer, supporters and more, and more, opponents of paraprofessionals' employment.

## THE PARAPROFESSIONAL AND INSTITUTIONS OF HIGHER LEARNING

It is conceivable that a full employment human service society could be developed and that the services could attain high standards and an organized political constituency to insure continued support and, at the same time, race, class, and sex bias could continue as parts of the social structure. For paraprofessionals to be offered equal chances to become first class citizens in the world of the human services, they must have access to pertinent education. That can only happen with a true new career orientation; universities have been increasingly reluctant to move in that direction. Anything short of that, the author believes, will maintain differential treatment and could, in time produce serious instabilities in our society. This ultimately would lead to disagreements about the quality of service and even to confrontations and disruptions.

Any new experimentation in working and higher education must involve established universities whose efforts must be carefully evaluated. Only when universities break out of long established molds and become accessible and accountable, will it be possible to break with the unfortunate traditions of the past.

In this context, the ability to insure that persons starting at any place in the system can continue to advance to the upper rungs is of utmost importance. The youth working as an escort for senior citizens in a public transit system must be able to see the next career step and a logical way to get there. Otherwise, he/she has little to invest in what is otherwise just a menial job.

History teaches us that societies that couldn't grow, died. It is the ability to progress from one place to another that stamps a society. It is also this capability that will determine the paraprofessional's future.

### REFERENCES

Bassett, T. R. *Education for the individual: A humanistic introduction,* New York: Harper and Row, 1978, pp. 107-108.

Fishman, S. et al. *The Community Apprentice Program,* Department of Health, Education and Welfare, Washington, D.C., 1965.

Friere, P. *The pedagogy of the oppressed,* New York: Harder and Harder, 1970.

Grant, J. D., & Grant, J. New careers development project: Final report, Unpublished manuscript, Institute for Study of Crime and Delinquency, Sacramento, Calif., 1967.

Grant, J. D., & Grant, J. Evaluation of New Career Programs. In *Handbook of the evaluation research,*

(Eds.). M. Guttentag and E. Struening, Beverly Hills, Calif.: Sage Publications, 1975.

Harrington, M. *The other america: Poverty in the United States.* New York: MacMillan, 1962.

Jones, M. et al., *The therapeutic community: A new treatment method in psychiatry.* New York: Basic Books, 1953.

McCorkle, L. W., Elias, A., & Bixby, F. L. *The Highfields story, a unique experiment in the treatment of juvenile delinquency.* New York: Holt, Rinehart and Winston, 1958.

Mayer, M. *The schools,* Garden City, New York: Doubleday 1961, p. 41.

Park, C. et al. The Bay City, Michigan experiment: A cooperative study for better utilization of teacher competence. (Symposium) *Journal of Teacher Education,* June 7, 1956, pp. 99-153.

Pearl, A., & Riessman, F. *New careers for the poor,* New York: Free Press (MacMillan), 1965.

Riessman, F., Kohler, M., & Gartner, A. *Children teach children,* New York: Harper and Row, 1971.

Riessman, F., Cohen, J., & Pearl, A. *Mental health of the poor,* New York: Free Press (MacMillan), 1964.

Sherif, M., & Sherif, C. Youth in lower class settings. In *Problems of youth,* Chicago: Aldine Press, 1965.

Theobald, R. *Guaranteed Income; The Next Step in Economic Evaluation,* New York: Doubleday, 1964.

U.S. Department of Commerce, Bureau of the Census. Statistical Abstract of the United States, 1977.

# Paraprofessionals: Past, Present and Future

Alan Gartner,
*Center for Advanced Study in Education,
City University of New York*

The United States is a country of fads—the à la mode, today's "hot" topic. When a new development is no longer media "sexy" (and few things stay that way for very long), one is normally inclined to believe that it has disappeared. On the other hand, it may be that the new has become part of the old, not gone, but no longer separate. It is the author's contention that, for the most part, this is what has happened to the paraprofessional.

In many ways, the paraprofessional is now a part of the fabric of the human services, distinct in some manner, but not detached. This holds mixed consequence. Before we assess them, however, the phenomena should be examined.

More than half of the personnel in mental health are paraprofessionals.

In the recent retrenchment of staff in the New York City Public Schools, the percentage of paraprofessionals discharged was no greater than that of the teachers.

At the heart of President Carter's welfare proposal is the creation of more than one million paraprofessional jobs in the human services.

In a review of the literature regarding mental health providers other than professionals, Gershon and Biller, 1977, cite more than 1,000 books, articles, and reports about paraprofessionals. A study for the Paraprofessional Branch of the National Institute of Mental Health (NIMH) reports an even greater number of citations (Alley et al., 1977a).

Thus, in areas where the work force is stable, declining, or potentially increasing, paraprofessionals are so much a part of the fabric of services, that they are no longer exceptional. Too much, of course, can be made of this; indeed, we will assert in the following pages that in many ways paraprofessionals are different and their contribution can be special. It is important to see, however, the paraprofessional role today for what it is now and not retain the context of the early 1960s. At that time paraprofessionals' were introduced into the human services on a large scale basis. It is a mistake to believe that paraprofessionals are no longer relevant.

## THE HUMAN SERVICES NEED

Although the traditional services in education, mental health, safety, social services, etc. are severely (and often rightly) deprecated as ineffective and expensive, nevertheless, there remains continued pressure for the expansion of all kinds of services. Legislation now mandates that all handicapped and retarded children receive education; no longer can these children be ignored or left at home. Court decisions require that mental patients receive rehabilitative treatment; no longer can they simply be incarcerated. There is also great concern for the number of abused children with some using the label "epidemic."

A study at the height of the expansionist mood of the 1960s estimated the need for nearly 4 million jobs in various service sectors (Greenleigh Associates, 1965, p. 36). Its findings were as follows:

TABLE A

*Estimates of Public Service Employment "Needs"*

| Field of Service | Potential |
|---|---|
| Health, including mental health and hospital | 1,355,000 |
| Education | 2,016,900 |
| Day Care | 14,000 |
| Recreation and Beautification | 136,000 |
| Libraries | 62,700 |
| Public Welfare | 65,000 |
| Probation and Parole | 16,000 |
| Institutions, dependent and delinquent children | 38,500 |
| Public Works | 150,000 |
| Police and Fire | 50,000 |
| Prison | 24,000 |
| Total: | 3,930,100 |

A year later, from a somewhat different perspective, the "Automation Commission" estimated that more than 5 million jobs could be created through public service employment (National Commission . . . , 1966, Vol. 1, p. 120). Here is a breakdown of the Commission's assessments:

Estimates of Potential Sources of New Jobs
Through Public Service Employment

| Source of Employment | Job Potential |
|---|---|
| Medical institutions and health services | 1,200,000 |
| Educational institutions | 1,100,000 |
| National beautification | 1,300,000 |
| Welfare and home care | 700,000 |
| Public protection | 350,000 |
| Urban Renewal | 650,000 |
| Total: | 5,300,000 |

(An important activity would be to update these estimates in light of new needs and new conditions.)
With a quite different focus, that of jobs for welfare clients, the U.S. Department of Labor reports more than a million and a half job slots, two-thirds of them in human service work (U.S. Department of Labor, 1977).[1]

Major Categories of Job Creation

| Category | Total Estimate |
|---|---|
| Public Safety | 155,000 |
| Building and repairing recreational facilities | 221,500 |
| Creating facilities for the handicapped | 31,000 |
| Environmental monitoring | 59,300 |
| Child care | 168,000 |
| Waste treatment and recycling | 32,500 |
| Cleanup and pest control | 110,000 |
| Home services for the elderly and ill | 237,000 |
| Running recreational programs | 141,200 |
| Weatherization | 65,800 |
| Paraprofessionals in the schools | 160,000 |
| School facilities improvement | 128,000 |
| Cultural arts activities | 86,500 |
| Total | 1,599,300 |

Accompanying these figures, the Department of Labor

[1] The estimates are of jobs suited to the Administration's welfare reform purposes, that is the jobs involve low skill levels, can pay minimum wages, need not erode existing wage structures, and are in new or expanding areas where there is important work to be done. The purpose of citing these data here is not to argue the welfare reform issue, but to offer additional information as to paraprofessional job

gives examples of specific jobs in these areas, such as: patrolling high fire risk districts, conducting home inspections, and fire safety demonstrations; escorting senior citizens; providing traffic and crowd control; inspecting homes for security deficiencies and providing instruction in remedying security problems; working in preschool day care centers; caring for small groups of young children in home settings; supervising after-school study hours and playground activities of children whose parent(s) work; providing childcare in public offices where parents seek services; providing home services to the elderly and ill including preparing meals, performing household chores, delivering meals; providing links between the old and the community through visiting, scheduling appointments, providing transportation; screening for basic medical problems; developing and supervising recreation programs for young and old; performing as teacher aides; providing ombudsman services; working as museum aides, library aides, cultural outreach workers; staffing emergency ambulance services; counselling delinquent youth; outreach programs to inform people about benefits and services; conducting surveys to determine community needs; providing transportation services; and working to identify and help abused or neglected children.

Although the figures of the Greenleigh Associates, Automation Commission, and Department of Labor are estimates, the current Comprehensive Employment and Training Act (CETA) provides concrete examples of current ongoing paraprofessional human service work in communities throughout the United States. Some of them are:

Stark County, Ohio—organizing security patrols for the public housing authority;

---

opportunities. Given the criteria used in selection for welfare reform purposes, the totals here are but a part of the entire paraprofessional potential.

Massilon, Ohio—establishing security patrols in public parks;

Springfield, Mo.—day care and teachers aides in a program for working parents;

Battle Creek, Mich.—housekeeping aides provide services to senior citizens to enable them to maintain their own homes or apartments;

West Palm Beach, Fla.—"Chore Companions" to assist homebound disadvantaged;

Battle Creek, Mich.—establishing a recreational program for the handicapped;

Boston, Mass.—nutrition specialists based at a school serving children from low-income families;

Whitehall, Mich.—roving ombudspersons available in school and the community;

Oakland, Calif.—establishing art exhibits in various public buildings;

Wiliniar, Minn.—providing library services to the homebound and hospitalized;

Green Bay, Wis.—organizing a museum's film collection.

## PARAPROFESSIONAL WORK IN MENTAL HEALTH: AN EXAMPLE

In light of the 1975 legislative mandate requiring federally-supported Community Mental Health Centers (CMHCs) to provide 12 types of mental health services (inpatient, outpatient, emergency, daycare, consultation and education, follow-up, transitional, screening, alcohol abuse, drug abuse, and services specifically for children and the aging), the Paraprofessional Branch of NIMH, commissioned the Social Action Research Center to conduct a study of the utilization of paraprofessionals in each of these areas (Alley, et al., 1977b). They found paraprofessionals performing in all of the 12 areas. The following are some examples:

They constitute two-thirds of the staff (including the Center's director) of the Permian Basin Centers for Mental Health and Mental Retardation in Odessa Texas. Paraprofessionals provide all of the direct and indirect services to alcohol clients.

The psycho-social rehabilitation program for chronic patients at the Community Mental Health Center of the Rutgers, N.J. Medical School makes particular use of paraprofessionals in life-skills training.

In Project Eden, Haywood, Calif. most of the staff, including the director, are paraprofessionals. The paraprofessionals staff a residential program, emergency rescue services, a drop-in center, hot-line, counseling, drug education and prevention services, and an employment and training program for youthful non-addicted drug abusers.

A total of 14 of the 17 clinicians of the Southwest Denver Community Mental Services are paraprofessionals. They provide services in the community by seeing two-thirds of their clients in "natural settings," usually through home visits.

At the Mid Columbia, Wash. Community Mental Health Center, the inpatient unit provides short-term hospitalization and milieu therapy with primary day-to-day care provided by paraprofessionals and nurses.

Although it is rare for paraprofessionals to be used in screening services, the Roxbury, Mass. Court Clinic employs paraprofessionals in that capacity. Here, paraprofessionals are used to screen prisoners assigned by the court as well as to work in special drug and alcohol screening programs.

Although these six cases of effective programs are not unique, they do suggest something of the breadth of paraprofessional work in community mental health centers. In view of this, it is somewhat ironic to note that between 1970 and 1976, CMHCs increased their professional staffing by 17%, while paraprofessionals have declined by 15%.

It is not only the range of paraprofessionals' work that commands our attention, but the effectiveness of their performance which must provide the ultimate justification. In another chapter, in Paraprofessionals in Mental Health, the author has discussed performance data in mental health. [And elsewhere (Gartner, 1971), the author surveyed the data in several human services fields.]

Beyond effectiveness as paraprofessionals, there are now data that indicate the superior performance of teachers recruited from paraprofessional ranks and prepared in a New Careers design of training (Kaplan, 1977). A full discussion of the Career Opportunities Program (COP), where paraprofessional school workers were prepared to be teachers, is beyond the scope of focus here. The data from a careful study comparing the effectiveness as teachers of those recruited from the traditional sources and prepared in the traditional manner with persons from the paraprofessional ranks and participating in an education and training program built into their jobs (Costa, 1975), provides powerful evidence in support of the proposition that New Careerists will be new (and better) professionals. The testing of this in fields other than education would be an important activity.

## WHY PARAPROFESSIONALS?

In *New Careers for the Poor,* (1965), Pearl and Riessman enumerated three reasons for the development of New Careers Programs—to improve the quality of the services, to relieve professional shortages, and to offer employment and career opportunities to the poor. These continue to be valid, if not all inclusive bases for the employment of paraprofessionals. To a greater extent than Pearl and Riessman initially realized, however, the activities involved in the relief of professional shortages are at odds with other activities of paraprofessionals to improve the quality of services.

Most current paraprofessional activities can be seen as the result of "shredding" out from professionals' work some activities that the professional does not care to do or for which professional preparation (and salary costs) are not necessary. Then, there are those activities where some special attribute of the paraprofessional, particularly a characteristic shared with the consumer, such as age, sex, race, ethnicity, prior experience is seen as the basis for the work role. Finally, there are activities, often new to the field of practice, where either professionals have not yet gained hegemony (or do not care to) or where some characteristic of the paraprofessional especially suits the person to the work. Of course, there is overlapping among these three bases for the work which paraprofessionals do. Thus, for example, although outpatient work in mental health could be done by a psychiatrist, often a paraprofessional does it both because the professional may not care to be out in the community and the paraprofessional may have a special capability to work there.

Lack of clarity as to the primary basis of paraprofessional utilization in a given situation often is at the root of tension between the professional and the paraprofessional, and frequently leads to misuse of the professional. Where the paraprofessional's role derives from the corpus of professionals' work, where the paraprofessional is in truth a subprofessional (or sometimes a professional-in-training), the leadership of the professional is appropriate. On the other hand, there is human services work where the paraprofessional, in fact, is doing something quite different from work done by the professional. Looking at various types of practice, particularly the work of self-help mutual aid groups, natural support systems, and indigenous healers, the author and Frank Riessman (1977) have developed the concept of "aprofessional practice." Here, aprofessional practice is contrasted with the dimensions of professional practice:

Table B

| Professional | Aprofessional |
|---|---|
| 1. Emphasis on knowledge and insight, underlying principles, theory, and structures. | 1. Emphasis on feeling, affect-the concrete and practical |
| 2. Systematic | 2. Experience, common sense, and intuition are central; folk knowledge |
| 3. "Objective"—Use of distance and perspective, self-awareness, control of transference | 3. Closeness and self-involvement; subjective |
| 4. Empathy controlled warmth | 4. Identification |
| 5. Standardized performance | 5. Extemporaneous, spontaneous (expressions of own personality) |
| 6. Outside orientation | 6. Insider orientation; indigenous |
| 7. Praxis | 7. Practice |
| 8. Careful, limited use of time; systematic evaluation; curing | 8. Slow, time no issue; informal direct accountability; caring |

Of course, these comparisons represent ideal types and in many cases professional and aprofessional practice overlap. And, so, too, the paraprofessional even when in the role of "subprofessional" brings his or her personal characteristics which may affect the professionals' practice. It is essential to distinguish, however, the bases of using paraprofessionals and to develop strategies appropriate to them. Thus, for example, the line of hierarchy from A.A. level to B.A. to M.S.W. to A.C.S.W. may be appropriate where social work discipline is the core of the practice, but there is not a similar basis to assign a medicine man, with twelve to sixteen years of training, to a position subordinate to a psychologist in a mental health program serving American Indians.[2] In the former case, career ladders within the profession are needed; in the latter an alternative pattern is necessary.


## THE FUTURE

Just as there are several different types of paraprofessionals, so, too, there are several different directions for the future of paraprofessionalism. At one level, in the day-to-day operation of traditional services, paraprofessionals are established as part of the ongoing staffing—not as something special, simply routine. Second, if there is an expansion of public service employment programs, in connection with welfare reform or full employment, a significant portion of this expansion is likely to occur among human services paraprofessionals. So, too, as the area of human services itself expands, there is likely to be an increase of paraprofessional activity. Education of the handicapped, for example, is such a field (Fafard, 1974; Fafard, 1977; Fafard and Pickett, 1977; Pickett, 1977a; Pickett, 1977b). Third, as new forms of practice develop (or as old forms, such as natural support systems, gain new recognition) paraprofessionals as aprofessional practitioners will have an important role.

Our view, then, is not for a replay of the 1960s, but rather a new set of developments, building upon the earlier period, but in many ways vastly more interesting.

The nature of these future developments may be seen in looking at a particular field. While there are several areas where marked developments as affects paraprofessionals are taking place—for example in day care, home health programs, education for the handicapped—the

[2]See, Indigenous Mental Health Paraprofessionals on an Indian Reservation, Kahn, et al., in the volume (editors' note).

mental health field offers the best illustration, in part, at least, because of the recent attention through the work of The President's Commission on Mental Health (The President's Commission on Mental Health, 1978).

The Commission took a broad view of mental health, as did its Task Panel on Personnel. They identified a number of broad trends affecting the overall human services, as well as the mental health field (The President's Commission on Mental Health, 1978, Vol. 2, pp. 424-425): the trend to deinstitutionalization and the development of community based services; the trend to the development of self-help groups and renewed interest in natural systems of support in neighborhoods and communities (churches, friends, lodges, etc.); the trend to greater interdependence of these stages as they all work with multiproblem persons and families in the communities; the trend to the sharing not only of the same kinds of personnel, but even of the same persons over a period of time; the trend to innovative service delivery programs; the trend to preventive activities and the promotion of wellbeing in addition to remedial and supportive services; and trends to demand accountability in terms of cost control, productivity, and quality assurance.

Each of these trends involves and has consequence for paraprofessionals.

The Commission's *Report* summarizes the developments in the paraprofessional field.

> In many ways the category of paraprofessionals is a catch-all. Until the past 10 years, there were few middle level workers in the mental health delivery system. Psychiatric aides were persons who had no training for their largely custodial jobs in institutions and no status in the system. They were given brief inservice training to provide basic nursing care, surveillance of wards, and housekeeping, and escort services.

However, under the impetus of the civil rights movement and the New Careers movement there began to be established a number of programs to train and employ mental health workers at middle levels. Many of these workers were hired as part of the new careers movement and trained in agency based programs of relatively short duration (3-6 months). Others were trained in technical institutes or community colleges where they received associate degrees. Altogether, more than over 500 such programs have trained over 30,000 such workers. A few are trained in baccalaureate programs to prepare mental health/human service workers. The development of training programs has been largely a local initiative that has been responsive to local needs rather than to any coordinated national initiative, although the New Careers program of the Federal Government provided impetus for the "hire now-train later" movement for all of the human services. The NIMH provided grant assistance to a variety of experimental training programs in the early 1960s, and in the late 1960s there were several time-limited developmental grants to a number of 2-year training programs in community colleges or in 4-year colleges. Then in 1970, NIMH created the New Careers Branch which became the Paraprofessional Manpower Development Branch in 1975. This program has concentrated on developing curriculum guidelines, studies of employment patterns, issues in credentialing, etc., more than on the ongoing funding of training. [It is noteworthy that the Branch's Director, Vernon James, was a participant in one of the first "New Careers" programs.]

The Southern Regional Education Board recently conducted a national survey that identified 354 paraprofessional training programs—more than over 200 in community colleges or 4-year colleges. The graduates of these associate degree programs have increased from 4,000 in the year 1970 to 10,000 per year in 1977 and are projected to be 12,500 per year in 1980.

The statistics regarding the staffing of mental health facilities show that 45 percent of all the full-time equivalent patient care staff had less than a BA degree, and this total comprises 130,000 mental health workers. This includes psychiatric aides, mental health technicians, and a number of other job titles; indeed, one of the difficulties in classifying these workers is that they tend to be titled by functional job titles rather than by any overall occupational title. Over 90 percent of these paraprofessionals working in mental health facilities are employed in inpatient settings.

Surveys of the work of paraprofessionals, however, show that they work in virtually every kind of mental health setting from mental hospital to community outreach and aftercare. They work with clients of all ages, and with all kinds of disorders, and studies show that they are effective in their therapeutic work with many clients. (pp. 441-442)

This background forms the base for a set of impressive recommendations by the Task Panel (pp. 473-475).

## PARAPROFESSIONAL PERSONNEL

The entire area of the development of middle level workers (paraprofessionals) is new and requires stronger federal and national definition and leadership. Much of the present system has grown in response to local needs and issues rather than from any national leadership. There is more need for definition and integration of these workers into the personnel system than support for training programs themselves.

## Recommendation

The NIMH and other Federal manpower programs should strengthen efforts to define and integrate the paraprofessional movement in the mental health delivery system. There are several sub-items:
A.  The funding of the Paraprofessional Manpower Development Branch of NIMH should be increased to better recognize the size of the paraprofessional personnel component of the mental health delivery system.

These workers comprise almost half of the personnel component. The funding authority should be for both grants and contracts to a variety of educational institutions: mental health agencies, and other organizations primarily for research and development of the various aspects of the credentialing, education, utilization, and evaluation of paraprofessionals and indigenous mental health professionals.
B.  The ADAMHA and other Federal agencies should initiate efforts in-house and with contracts and grants to develop a coordinated conceptualization of the role and functions of paraprofessional workers and their relationships to the paraprofessionals and their clients.

Because the paraprofessional movement has grown from many different local initiatives, there is presently a somewhat confusing welter of levels, roles, titles, training programs, and career systems.

Some specific issues to address are:
1.  The development of a set of definitions of terms that can be generally accepted in the field.
2.  Further exploration and definition of the role of a generic Human Services Worker.

3.  Definition of the various levels in a career system for paraprofessionals in mental health delivery programs.
4.  Further exploration and definition of the appropriate roles and functions for various models of paraprofessionals.
5.  The development of guidelines for the utilization of paraprofessionals vis-à-vis the existing professionals in various team models, staff structures, and supervisory relationships. This kind of information needs to be included in the continuing education and the pre-professional training of the professionals as well.

C.  Paraprofessional Manpower Development Branch and other components of ADAMHA should pursue efforts to define an appropriate credentialing program for paraprofessionals. The possession of credentials promotes recognition of skills and facilities both geographic and interagency mobility.

D.  NIMH, NIDA, and NIAAA should encourage further studies and guidelines for competency based approaches to training and credentialing of paraprofessionals.

The paraprofessional programs have already done considerable work in this area which promises to develop more efficient approaches to training and worker assessment for actual service delivery.

E.  NIMH should encourage the development of guidelines and training materials for the training of paraprofessionals in specialty areas such as:
1.  child mental health;
2.  mental health of the aging; including the training of older paraprofessionals;
3.  prevention;
4.  work with self-help groups and community support programs; and;

     5.   relocation of institutional workers for community service work as institutional jobs are phased out.

F.   NIMH should support the development of linkages between the training programs for paraprofessionals and those for the professionals to assure that persons who wish to move up in academic careers can do so with a minimum of lost time, lost academic credits, and money.

This requires credit transfer arrangements, methods for assessing competence developed from experience, and curriculum linkages. The professional schools should recognize the paraprofessionals as a rich potential resource for the recruitment of motivated and experienced candidates, many of whom are minority persons.

G.   The ADAMHA and NIMH should include representation of the paraprofessionals and indigenous mental health practitioners on any advisory committees related to personnel, services, or data for which the inputs of the professions is deemed important.

There has been a tendency to recognize the professions only in the various advisory councils and committees. The paraprofessionals and indigenous mental health practitioners, although very diverse in function and training, should also be represented as they have substantial inputs to make into deliberations.

As the paraprofessional effort continues, there are dangers that must be recognized and countered.

1.   The new paraprofessional may be socialized by the professional without influencing the latter very much; in other words, instead of having cross-socialization in which both parties are affected, the impact may be largely one way, and the paraprofessional, moving up a career ladder may, by the time he or she arrives at professional status, be a replica of the old professional.

2. Movement up the ladder may not occur and large numbers of paraprofessionals may only be impacted at the bottom. There may be ladders with steps that do not reach beyond a very low point; thus, we may have family health aide worker 1, 2, 3, etc., without a new route for moving higher and breaking the credential barrier.

3. The efficiency of the human service system may be increased by the addition of the new personnel but not really reorganized so that professionals really perform essentially the same function as they did before only with more hands assisting them.

4. In moving from an overly-academic abstract, removed training model, there is the danger that the pendulum will swing too far in the other direction so that the workers will be trained largely in a simple type of on-the-job training where they will learn how to perform specific functions but not really be educated with systematic knowledge of a professional kind.

5. Paraprofessionals may be co-opted as a buffer to the community rather than being permitted to assist in changing the human service and professional systems.

6. Paraprofessionals may be utilized to substitute for, and compete with, professionals in order to save money for agencies.

7. The paraprofessionals may be "compartmentalized," separated off from the professionals, presumably to safeguard their identity, but the effect, of course, will be to limit their effect on the professionals as well as to impact them at the bottom of the ladder.

To counter these dangers, paraprofessionals (and their supporters) can look to at least four overlapping strategies to affect the profession and its practice.

*Strategy I.* Paraprofessionals may affect professionals

by working alongside them, changing the atmosphere of their agencies, sensitizing them to demands of the community as well as by participating in professional organizations and unions.

*Strategy II.* As paraprofessionals move up a career ladder to become professionals via new combinations of training, work and education, they may become a different kind of professional at the end of the route. In addition, as paraprofessionals the latter have the opportunity of performing new kinds of functions, e.g., consultation, supervision, training, management, administration, diagnosis.

*Strategy III.* Paraprofessionals may change professional practice by performing new work, new job functions such as health advocate, expediter, parent educator, program developer, thus providing a whole range of new human service practice.

*Strategy IV.* Paraprofessionals, in a variety of ways, may improve the performance, efficiency, productivity of human service agencies, and in so doing affect the professions.

For whatever else it is that the paraprofessional does, it is this last, the doing well in practice, that provides the firmest justification for their utilization, and indeed, expansion of their services. Addressing these items, no less meeting each of them, present a full agenda for the future of paraprofessionals.[3] Although they are likely to lack the sanction of a Presidential Commission, there is a similar array of future issues for paraprofessionals across the entire range of the human services.

---

[3]The NIMH Paraprofessional Branch has taken a new step to accelerate these development with the support of a national clearinghouse concerning paraprofessionals in mental health to be operated jointly by the New Careers Training Laboratory, Graduate School and University Center, City University of New York, and the Social Action Research Center, Berkeley, Calif.

REFERENCES

Alley, S., et al. *Paraprofessionals in mental health: An annotated bibliography from 1966 to 1977.* Berkeley, Calif.; Social Action Research Center, 1977a.

Alley, S., et al. *Paraprofessionals in mental health: Twelve effective programs.* Berkeley, Calif.; Social Action Research Center, 1977b.

Costa, C. *A comparative study of Career Opportunities Program graduates as teachers.* New York: New Careers Training Laboratory, 1975.

Fafard, M. *The utilization and training of paraprofessionals in special education: Present status and future prospects.* New York: New Careers Training Laboratory, 1974.

Fafard, M. *Paraprofessional movement in special education: Historical perspective.* New York: New Careers Training Laboratory, 1977.

Fafard, M., and Pickett, A. L. *Training of paraprofessionals in special education: Selected bibliography.* New York: New Careers Training Laboratory, 1977.

Gartner, A. *Paraprofessionals and their performance.* New York: Praeger Publishers, 1971.

Gartner, A., & Riessman, F. *Self-help in the human services.* San Francisco: Jossey-Bass, 1977.

Gershon, M., & Biller, H. B. *The other helpers: Paraprofessionals and non-professionals in mental health.* Lexington, Mass.: Lexington Books, 1977.

Greenleigh Associates. *A public employment program for unemployed poor.* New York, 1965.

Kaplan, G. *From aide to teacher; The story of the Career Opportunities Program.* Washington, D.C.: U.S. Government Printing Office, 1977.

National Commission on Technology, Automation and Economic Progress. *Technology and the American economy.* Washington, D.C.: U.S. Government Printing Office, 1966.

Pearl, A., and Riessman, F. *New careers for the poor.* New York: Free Press, 1965.

Pickett, A. L. *The training of paraprofessionals in special education: Results of a survey of institutions of higher education and descriptions of training programs.* New York: New Careers Training Laboratory, 1977a.

Pickett, A. L. *The utilization and training of paraprofessionals in special education: Results of a survey of state directors of special education and descriptions of training programs.* New York: New Careers Training Laboratory, 1977b.

President's Commission on Mental Health. *Report to the President from the President's Commission on Mental Health.* Washington, D.C.: Superintendent of Documents, 1978, Vols. 1-14.

U.S. Department of Labor. *Attachment on subsidized public service jobs and training.* Washington, D.C.: U.S. Department of Labor, August 6, 1977.

# The Economics of
# Paraprofessional Employment

Mark A. Haskell,
*College of Urban Affairs & Public Policy,*
*University of Delaware*

## THE ECONOMIC PERSPECTIVE

The scientific study of economics centers on two problems. The first concerns "allocation" or, more simply, why a society produces a particular mix of goods and services. The second has to do with "distribution," i.e., why the claims to these goods and services vary as they do. Taken together, these two areas constitute "microeconomics," the study of decision making by the individual, the household, and the business firm. Another major area, "macroeconomics," examines the long term performance of economic systems concentrating on economic stability, i.e., the aggregate levels of resource employment, and on economic growth over time.

From the standpoint of the overall performance of the economy, paraprofessional programs are a part of a large policy "menu" of programs aimed at achieving full employment. Some of these, such as monetary and fiscal policy, attempt to stimulate aggregate demand indirectly. Others, such as public service employment, increase demand for labor directly through federal appropriation of funds for that purpose.

On the other hand, all training activities including paraprofessional training assume adequacy of overall demand for labor, with a mismatch between the supply of particular skills and the demand for those responsible for unemployment above a "frictional" level. The aim of such programs is a qualitative alteration of skills to realign them with the needs of the labor market.

National economic policy under three administrations, however, has decreed a relatively high level of unemployment as hostage against greater inflation, leaving the success of any training program problematic. The national unemployment rate was six percent or greater for almost four years from October 1974, falling to 5.7 percent in June 1978. Annual averages were 8.5 percent in 1975, 7.7 percent in 1976, 7.0 percent in 1977, and 6.0 percent in 1978, with a high of 8.9 percent in May 1975.[1] The current unemployment rate (July 1979) is 5.7 percent but the Carter administration expects it to increase to 6.6 percent by the end of 1979 and to 8.2 percent by November 1980 (New York Times, 1979). These rates have consistently been among the highest in the industrialized world. Clearly the assumption of adequate aggregate demand for labor is not valid, especially when one considers the extremely high incidence of unemployment

[1]The drop in the unemployment rate from 7.0% in November, 1977 to 6.4% in December, the lowest rate since October, 1974 seems in large part due to a revision in the method used to calculate unemployment.

among minorities and young persons. For blacks and other minorities, joblessness is almost 11 percent; for persons 16 to 19 years of age, it is above 13 percent for whites and near 31 percent for blacks (U.S. Bureau of Labor Statistics, 1979).

In the microeconomic tradition, the economic analysis of paraprofessional employment is a subset of the analysis of public expenditure, that, in turn, is thoroughly grounded in microeconomics. For economists, however, the economics of the public sector presents a serious dilemma. Many are content to let individual decisions determine allocation and distribution in the private sector and, in fact, claim that the sum of such decisions leads to the most optimal outcomes. In the public sector, no such impersonal mechanism is present; all choices are conscious ones made through a political process. In large part then, the development of the economics of the public sector has been a search for mechanisms which can reasonably replicate the private sector and a search for tools of analysis that can determine whether or not that goal has been accomplished.

## Cost-Benefit Analysis

For economists, the tool of choice in the evaluation of public programs has been cost-benefit analysis, a method of estimating whether the returns generated by a particular public program are adequate to justify its cost, and adequate to justify its choice over alternative programs or over no program at all.[2]

---

[2]Cost-benefit analysis is distinguished from cost-effectiveness analysis in that both program costs and benefits in the former are expressed in money terms. In the latter, benefits are expressed as direct program outputs and no attempt is made to give them a market value. Hence, an output such as improved student achievement is measured against the dollar cost of producing it. Here one cannot determine whether the benefits are greater than the costs, but the relative efficiency of two or more programs that have the same goal can be compared.

This technique has had widespread use in public sector economics and there are numerous examples of its application in government manpower programs. Somewhat strangely, however, its application to paraprofessional programs has been limited, although there is no intrinsic reason that this should be the case. A reasonable explanation is that the evaluation of paraprofessional programs has been dominated by noneconomists—sociologists, psychologists, social workers, and others whose concerns lie more in the areas of human development and improvement of service delivery than in an analysis of program cost factors. In such studies, questions of cost are rarely taken into account and where policy recommendations are made, it is usually assumed that if a group is performing well, more paraprofessional training in that field is justified. An economist would not accept such a conclusion—he/she would want to know whether the resources being committed might be more productive in some other use and would suggest that cost-benefit analysis of alternatives could provide a useful guide. Although that point should be granted, it is also true that cost-benefit analysis of paraprofessional training programs has very serious limitations; it is desirable that these limitations be made explicit.

## HUMAN CAPITAL THEORY AND ITS ALTERNATIVES

It is perhaps best to begin with the theoretical base for the technique, namely, human capital theory. This theory posits that increased education and training enhances human productivity directly and, hence, is a major cause of increased employability and earning power on that part of those who invest in it. Evidence that the theory has validity is shown by the positive correlation between education-training and income and by the negative correlation with unemployment rates.

Berg (1971) and others, however, have raised serious

questions about how much education and training do, in fact, increase human productivity. The critics argue that the principal output of much education and training is a "credential" that allows access to certain occupations and that job skills, themselves, are most often developed after the job has been obtained. Thurow's (1975) "job competition theory" is another version of this approach and the "dual labor market" theory (Doeringer and Piore, 1974) is a complementary attack on "human capital." The dual labor market theory questions that labor markets are characterized by reasonably open access to the higher rungs of the occupational ladder. The theory posits two distinct markets differing fundamentally from one another. In the primary market where there are high wages and good benefits, job security, favorable working conditions, and career ladders, human capital theory does apply. In the secondary labor market, however, where wages are low, jobs are dead-end, security is nil, unemployment is common, and work is intermittent and irregular, it most definitely does not. Here, workers are caught in a vicious cycle. Under these conditions, attitudes and behavior of workers are adversely affected and employers adjust their expectations to them; in fact they are said to encourage undisciplined behavior so as to freeze wages at minimum levels. Once in the secondary labor market, a worker finds it difficult to leave. If female or nonwhite, as a disproportionate number of secondary workers are, discrimination is a barrier; in any case, secondary market work habits may mitigate against opportunity to advance or may be the cause of failure if entry into the primary market is achieved.

For the paraprofessional, existence of a primary-secondary dichotomy is indicated by the persistence of credentialism (Grosser, 1969; Rosen, 1970). This is one of the important factors that may account for the difficulty that paraprofessionals encounter in advancing to professional positions. Evidence that upward mobility is a serious problem has support from recent research (Nixon,

Note 1; Brecher, 1972; Pointer, Note 2; Cleckley, Note 3; Cohen, 1976). That the existence of dual markets is beneficial to employers is suggested by Pearl (1974, p. 264), who charges that "paraprofessionals gained a measure of support from traditionally conservative politicians and administrators because they were cheap—cheap not only in wages but also in the ease with which they could be removed."

The implications of the contrasting theories are most significant for public policy. Human capital theory strongly implies that the cause of low income is in individual educational deficiencies or, simply, a matter of choice. Hence, the remedy for low income lies with the individual. On the other hand, the critics argue that the structure of the socioeconomic system lies at the heart of income disparity, and structural corrections are required to assure fair access to jobs to achieve improved income distribution. They further assert that the economic system cannot produce full employment without significant government intervention and that short of it, the labor market develops mechanisms to ration access to good jobs, career ladders and high incomes.

For manpower programs, the implications are clear. Where there are job shortages, those who enter the programs may be a chosen few who are being allowed some escape routes from unemployment or from the secondary labor market. When the training is for occupations where there are few new openings, the program may be a co-optation device or a temporary income maintenance scheme. Thurow (1972) agrees:

> If macroeconomic policies are being set in terms of target unemployment rates (as they were in the Kennedy-Johnson administration and are in the Nixon administration), every training program is simply a program for reshuffling employment or unemployment and not a program for reducing employment. (p. 253)

Recognizing the deficiencies of the theoretical base, it is still not unreasonable to state that many training programs do have significant effects on human skills and that cost-benefit analysis can assist us in targeting the limited government funds that are available to finance them. Hence, it is useful to point out the weaknesses of cost benefit analysis as a tool, quite apart from the global debate over conventional labor market theory, human capital theory, and the alternatives.

## TECHNICAL PROBLEMS OF COST-BENEFIT ANALYSIS

The major internal problems with cost-benefit analysis have to do with the availability of data and with its measurability in money terms.

The question of availability of data falls into three parts: 1) the availability of control groups; 2) measuring costs; and 3) measuring benefits. Since most analysts believe that a "before and after" analysis cannot adequately isolate the effect of the program itself from non-program influences on the individual, it is necessary to have a non-trained control group with which to compare the trainees. In the vast majority of programs, given legislative and administrative necessity, programs have been put in place prior to any thought of systematic evaluation. Hence, most cost-benefit studies have had of necessity to take the "before and after" form and must, therefore, be considered methodologically deficient.

On the cost side, the most gross estimate that has to be made is the calculation of opportunity costs; that is, earnings that are foregone by the trainee in order to undertake the program and enter into a new career. The significance of this cannot be overstated—human capital theory assumes that this calculation can be made with some exactitude. Consequently, it is very difficult to measure this loss and great inaccuracy can be assumed. Moreover, there is often difficulty in capturing the actual cost of a given program from government records. This is particularly problematic where there are "joint-costs;" that is, where particular personnel or a particular facility are used in more than one program.

But whatever the difficulties with cost estimation, the benefit side clearly presents far greater mysteries. The benefits of a program can be very widespread; hence, there is a problem in tracing them. Moreover, some are readily measurable in money terms; at the other extreme, any attempt at conversion to money terms is sheer guesswork.

The measurement problem is simplest where *individual* benefits are concerned. These are increases in earnings and additional fringe benefits, as well as an expected reduction in the incidence of unemployment. The latter presents obvious problems, but even the estimate of the former is not so simple as it may seem. Depending on occupation, it is somewhat hazardous to predict future earnings as most program evaluations are completed a relatively short time after training has been finished.

At the level of benefits to *government,* the measurement problem is more complicated, but not insoluble. Here, the problem is to estimate increases in taxes from participants and others, and decreases in spending on transfer payments or on crime and public safety, if any. The next set of benefits are those which accrue to *society* at large and it is here that the measurement problem becomes very sticky. Most of these benefits are quite indirect, such as increases in income to others due to tax reductions and derived increases in productivity or the political benefits of more equity. In either case, whether the benefits are economic or noneconomic, measurement tends to take on a very subjective quality.

## COST-BENEFIT: AN ILLUSTRATION

One of the few "pure" economic evaluations of a paraprofessional program does illustrate very well the contributions and limitations of cost-benefit analysis. This study, Scheffler's analysis of physician's assistants (PA) programs, concentrates strictly on the *private* benefits of such training. The purpose of the study was to determine the private rate of return to training and was based on a mail survey of all graduates of physician's assistants programs between 1967 and 1972. The major conclusions are that (1975, p. 79) " . . . the private rate of return is sufficient to produce a relatively strong demand for PA training:" and " . . . therefore, an increase in government support to trainees appears to be unwarranted." Specifically, rates of return, considering both direct and indirect costs of training are found to be close to 20%, varying with assumed discount rates and rates of growth of income.

Scheffler's paper is replete with the esoterica of modern econometrics and mathematical economics. Hence, he deals with opportunity costs, discount rates, makes estimates for missing data and for growth of income, all in the context of a multiple regression model. An economist, trained to do cost-benefit studies, would have little to quarrel with in this careful, conventional effort.

Nonetheless, however strong in methodology, the weaknesses of the study are multifarious in terms of policy. These weaknesses stem directly from the limitations of cost-benefit analysis discussed earlier. For example, the conclusion that government support of PA programs should not be increased[3] is based solely on the assumption that 20% rate of return on investment is sufficient to induce adequate numbers of persons to undergo training. No explanation is provided; economists simply assume that a relatively free market will bring supply of PAs into balance with demand.

Two major problems are apparent here. On the supply side, the policy conclusion overlooks the fact that private

[3]The author (p. 79) suggests that support might even be reduced.

financing, either personal or through financial institutions, is usually not available to low income persons; hence, the freezing or reduction of government support could effectively limit entry to the program for many of them. With respect to demand, no account is taken of the need for health services on the part of persons who cannot afford them; in the jargon of economists, they evince no "effective demand." When these matters are taken into consideration, it is far from an obvious conclusion that a given private rate of return to training will provide society with all of the physician's assistants it needs, which is, in effect, the conclusion that the author does offer.

Even within the logic of cost-benefit, if the author had considered benefits to government or benefits to society at large, the conclusion might have been different. For government, more funds devoted to this program might be offset by reduced amounts devoted to the construction of medical schools and subsidies for their operation. For society, the benefit of improved health care in areas with insufficient numbers of physicians might justify enlargement of the program.

Other criticisms can be made. Scheffler neglects the possibility that paraprofessionals might have a special contribution to make to health care in low income or in ethnic enclaves. The model is strictly along engineering or "job factoring" lines with PAs simply performing routine work not requiring the skills of fully-qualified practitioners; the new careers model is overlooked. Also, the effect on the low income population in terms of positive role models and increased incentive for school completion is ignored.

In short, the author did his technical analysis very well; the finding that graduates of PA programs fare well economically is a significant and useful one. Also of significance for policy are the findings regarding the differences in earnings resulting from background characteristics and from program specialties. Nonetheless, the author was unable to relate his analysis through policy conclusions to the real world of health service delivery, imperfect markets, inequality, and poverty. What the study lacks most is an analysis of the special contributions physician's assistant might be able to make; a discussion of real medical need, as opposed to simple economic demand for these services; and a recognition of fuller socioeconomic implications of the program.

Some of these considerations are, in fact, dealt with by Walker (Note 4) in her study of the supply of labor for paramedical occupations. While she concludes that private rates of return on training investments are "attractive," she points out that limited mobility and inadequate information on the availability of training opportunities and their costs and benefits are serious constraints affecting the possibility of securing adequate numbers of trainees in the three occupations—licensed vocational nursing, medical technology and inhalation therapy—that she studied.

## OTHER EVALUATION TECHNIQUES

Even at its best, cost-benefit analysis must be considered only one of several approaches to the evaluation of public programs. In addition to it, Hamermesh (1971, pp. 3-4) cites several other economic approaches to the study of manpower training. One in particular—that of going beyond the first order effects of programs and tracing them into the larger domestic or international economy —seems especially important. Here, aggregate variables such as national unemployment rates would be stressed as would changes in social indicators of education and health.

Barsby (1972, p. 7) suggests that cost-benefit analysis "merely suggests how well a program is operating when viewed in a specific way." Thus, he concludes that a multi-dimensional and multidisciplinary perspective must be used to provide the most useful evaluation. Non-economic analyses using observation, interviews and question-naires can focus on the internal operations of programs so as to disentangle the effective from the noneffective components and to hone in on the difficult questions of personality and community change and other psychosoci-ological consequences of manpower programs.

Economists have, in fact, been delinquent in this re-spect. In their comprehensive examination of manpower program evaluation, Perry et al. (1975) state that

> the voluminous literature on program evaluation re-viewed for this study offers very little evidence on the non-economic effects of training on program par-ticipants. Of the more than 200 studies included in the search for data, only 17 contained any informa-tion pertaining to program effects other than the impact upon employment and earnings. (pp. 93-94)

Such, obviously, has not been the case with respect to paraprofessional training where economic evaluations are rare. In the same volume, Matlack (1975, p. 216) cor-rectly points out that "the evaluative literature on the New Careers Program is subjective in nature, often em-phasizing the impact the program has on the delivery of services rather than the impact of the program on enrol-lees." Of course, the vast bulk of these evaluations are the products of non-economists who have tended to see New Careers as a broad social movement that could induce significant social change rather than simply as a man-power training program in the "human capital" tradi-tion. Economists have probably tended to ignore New Careers programs because in terms of resources commit-ted, they have been minuscule in relationship to such "giants" as MDTA and more recently CETA.

## Some Eclectic Evaluations

While less technically rigorous, other secondary and primary evaluations provide a more balanced perspective than does Scheffler's study. For example, Cohen's (1976a) recent study of paraprofessional experience provides a multi-dimensional perspective. It views: 1) the social and psychological effects of the programs on the paraprofessionals themselves; 2) the effect of the programs on service delivery; and 3) the effect on national manpower and service delivery policy.

Most evidence is forthcoming on the second question. On the basis of it, Cohen concludes (1976b, p. 7) that "properly trained, supervised, and supported paraprofessionals can be effective deliverers of human services." Regarding the effect on national policy, the conclusion is more negative; namely, that the larger objectives—social reform and institutional change have not been achieved in any substantial way (1976a, p. 105). This finding reinforces Grosser's (1969) widely quoted conclusion that "a useful and relevant, albeit limited, strategy" has been "inflated to the gradiose status of a social movement" (p. 6). Cohen grants that the New Careers strategy has been, almost exclusively, a technique by which some number of uncredentialed persons have been able to secure previously unattainable jobs and have performed satisfactorily, sometimes more satisfactorily than professionals.

Although the chapters on program and policy are detailed, the findings on economic effects are skimpy. The author establishes that post-program earnings have increased for paraprofessionals, but these increases have been largely dissipated through inflation. Salaries still hover, for the most part, on the poverty line, and upward mobility is found to have been extremely limited (1976a, p. 57).

Most other studies provide less than Cohen's on questions of economic efficiency. Reviewing 15 years of studies of paraprofessionals in guidance and counseling, Brown

(1974) finds numerous reports testifying to the effectiveness of their work, but faults most of them as being methodologically weak. For our purposes, it is enough to point out that none of them, including several done by Brown and associates, deal with questions of cost; the main focus is on the effectiveness of service delivery and on the reactions of professionals and clients to paraprofessionals.

Also in the field on counseling and community mental health, Hoffman and Warner (1976) surveyed 85 primary studies. Here, too, the question of service delivery effectiveness outweighs all other perspectives. Questions of economic efficiency are not dealt with at all, although the authors cite the need for "cost-effectiveness" studies (p. 496).

Another major "study of studies," the U.S. Department of Health, Education and Welfare's *Overview Study of Employment of Paraprofessionals* (1974), cites the same problem of the lack of rigorous, controlled research and finds that cost-effectiveness analysis was infrequently used (p. 105). The sole example cited compared a control group of two persons with a slightly larger experimental group and provided data only for the relative cost of service delivery (p. 105). The advantage of the experimental group in quality of service provided was not integrated into the cost figures.

Gartner's (1971) study of paraprofessional performance focuses on a number of fields—education, mental health, social work, health, police, corrections, and law enforcement. And while it views the impact of the paraprofessional on human services in a sensitive and insightful way, it devotes just two pages to the question of costs and benefits. The fault is not Gartner's—there are not enough studies to require more space. But, nonetheless, the author is somewhat skeptical that cost-benefit analysis can make much of a contribution to the evaluation of paraprofessional programs: "estimating dollar value of human service programs is, in some ways, little more than an exercise in more or less educated guessing" (p. 107). He goes on, however, to say that if such an analysis is " . . . done carefully and accepted with due caution, it can give some indication of the parameters of the issue" (p. 107).

A Senate Education and Labor Committee study cited by Gartner includes "direct social benefits from a public service job development program" (p. 107) as measured by increases in gross national product. Hence, benefits to the individual are coupled with increased benefits from public services. A second study, this of a Minneapolis New Careers program points out that there are significant benefits in addition to private ones. These include decreases in law enforcement and other public expenses and unspecified positive effects on family and friends of the trainee (p. 107). A third, an analysis of a program designed for juvenile offenders, cited three types of benefits: 1) reduced costs to the public due to the dropping of cases of juveniles participating in the program and as a result of a reduction in recidivism; 2) higher employment rates for participants; and 3) increased earnings and productivity of participants (p. 108).

Moving to actual field investigations, Conant's (1973) cost-effectiveness analysis of paraprofessionals in education is one of the more elaborate studies. It focuses particularly on two aspects of paraprofessionals in education: 1) changes in the " . . . kinds and amounts of instruction that are performed in the schools"; and 2) whether "the costs of this new work division (can) be justified in terms of student learning experiences and other benefits it may confer?" (p. xvii)

Overall, Conant judged the cost-effectiveness results to be "very favorable" (p. 64), although the failure of professional teachers to alter their work patterns very much clouds that conclusion.

Children received exceptional instruction only from

paraprofessionals whose employment costs were
borne by new expenditures of local, state, and federal funds. Newer, more effective instruction was
purchased for children, in effect, only by hiring non-
paraprofessionals to circumvent the traditional
teaching division of labor (p. 65).

This is reflected in the raw cost figures that showed a
substantial advantage in hourly teaching costs where
teacher and paraprofessional teams operated whether
this involved classroom or small group instruction. These
lower costs resulted from two effects: 1) professional
teachers providing more instruction time; and 2) added
paraprofessional instruction at a substantially lower
hourly wage. The latter was by far the most significant
element in the overall reduction of average hourly teaching costs since instructional hours were doubled when
paraprofessionals were paired with teachers. Of course,
the actual quality of paraprofessional teaching was not
measured, but the author shows that even if the quality
of paraprofessional teaching instruction is assumed to be
only 50% of professional instruction, a large cost advantage of $7.51 per hour for classroom instruction and
$21.62 for small group instruction remains (p. 75).

When actual output measures are considered, the
findings are reinforced. There is considerable evidence
presented to show that the improvement of reading test
scores of children in the program was significantly influenced by the compensatory program. These improvements were obtained at an annual increased operations
cost per pupil of $435; this represents a 67% increase over
expenditures in nonprogram schools.

Whether the improvements are worth the cost can only
be a matter of judgment. There is no real way to translate
them into dollar figures, hence it is not possible to com-
pute a rate of return as in cost-benefit analysis. This, of
course, is a weakness of a cost-effectiveness approach

where benefits cannot be expressed in money units as they are in cost benefit analysis.

Other nonmeasured or nonmeasurable outcomes were also said to be achieved. These included closer relationships between teachers and pupils, greater attention to behavioral problems, and others. Most, however, could not be quantified in a cost-benefit analysis, but could be incorporated into a cost-effectiveness approach.

## MACROECONOMIC INFLUENCES AND EFFECTS

Thus far, this paper has concentrated on the micro-level analyses of economists and of other social and behavioral scientists that have dominated the literature on manpower training and on paraprofessionalism as well. Perhaps these approaches were sufficient during the 1960s and early 1970s when unemployment rates were low. Now, there is a greater understanding of the fact that the fate of paraprofessional as well as other training programs is directly tied to the overall performance of the economic system. Cohen (1976a, p. 3), Gartner and Riessman (1974, p. 255) and Pearl (1974, p. 268) have all pointed out recently that the high levels of unemployment pervasive through the second Nixon, Ford, and Carter administrations have not only dampened enthusiasm for manpower training, but have made their success next to impossible due to increased competition for available jobs from more impressively-credentialed workers. Gartner and Riessman (1977) are undoubtedly correct when they state " . . . in order to have genuine new careers, we will have to have full employment. We cannot simply move people up unless there is a vast expansion of jobs, jobs that are likely to be created in the public sector." According to Cohen (1976b, p. 10), the problem for new careers and for paraprofessional programs has been aggravated by the transfer through the Public Employment Program (PEP) of the Emergency

Employment Act and through the Comprehensive Employment and Training Act (CETA) of manpower planning to state and local governments. In the face of heavy unemployment, these governments have effectively sacrificed the major components of paraprofessional employment—training, career development and improved service delivery in favor of immediate public employment.

While public service employment has importance in providing higher levels of income than government transfer programs, in alleviating the fiscal problems of state and local governments, and in upgrading skills and work patterns of disadvantaged workers, they provide only a small portion of the benefits that regular jobs do. In particular, lifetime career opportunities are absent, and the level of skill development is much lower. Further, more public service employment at, or near, the minimum wage does little to reduce the income disparities that characterize our economic structure. If we are to make more than a token improvement in the employment situation, the answer must be found in expanding opportunities for unsubsidized employment whether this employment be along new careers lines or in more conventional modes.

Although full employment may be a necessary condition for the success of manpower programs, Pearl and Cohen are not convinced that it is necessarily a sufficient condition. Although Cohen (1976a, p. 109) calls for a drastic overhaul of human service delivery systems to compensate for " . . . lack of political power, insufficient resources, and fragmentated and uncoordinated patterns of service delivery . . . ," Pearl's requirements are more fundamental and his pessimism more obvious. Hence, "the concentration of wealth and power in the hands of a few requires that there be poverty, racism, dehumanized bureaucracy, warped priorities, alienation, feelings of impotence among the vast majority" (p. 266), and "calls for employing paraprofessionals up career ladders are empty without a change in the economy—a change that would markedly shift the emphasis from the manufacture of goods and the expenditure of energy to an emphasis on health, education, welfare, and other human services . . . " (p. 268).

But that kind of structural change can only be the evolutionary result of several strategies aimed at developing the political and economic potential of low income communities. Along these lines, perhaps the most efficacious policy prescriptions have been developed by a group of scholars who have rejected the once popular "suburbanization strategy" for disadvantaged groups. Vietorisz and Harrison (1971), for example, take a comprehensive view of "ghetto development" defining it as "an overall social and economic transformation, with a large increase in the diversity of higher economic and institutional functions which ghetto residents are capable of sustaining, matched by a decisive improvement in the cohesion of the ghetto community." They go on to envisage

> . . . the creation of a number of 'inside jobs,' acquisition by the community of assets both inside and outside the ghetto, a substantial expansion of existing black businesses (particularly through cooperative forms of ownership), the large-scale transfer of ghetto property to ghetto residents and/or the community *qua* community, emphasis on the provision of pre-vocational and skill training within these ghetto enterprises, and local control of community political institutions, e.g., schools, police, and health facilities. (pp. 29-30)

The emphasis on the importance of cooperative enterprises or on community development corporations owned by a neighborhood stems more from the potential for development of organizational skills and political power than from economic potential alone. The latter can be the product of more conventional forms of development, but those are likely to stifle the former. For Vietorisz and Harrison (1970), ghetto development is

> . . . far more than a mechanism for allocating re-
> sources efficiently, organizing production, generat-
> ing profit streams, or even creating jobs . . . Eco-
> nomic development . . . acts as a catalyst of social
> and political change. Jobs created inside the ghetto
> are the instruments as well as the objects of this
> change, contributing to a reduction in psychological
> and social pathology, an improvement in the 'tech-
> nology' of community organization, increased skill
> levels, and re-enforcement of the community's politi-
> cal base and potential. (p. 66)

In the ghetto development literature, the concept most akin to paraprofessionalism is that of "greenhouse industries" that are designed to break even, but which have as one of their main goals, the training of workers in a famil-
iar and sympathetic environment. In this program, one aim is to create the conditions under which workers can move into jobs outside the ghetto (Vietorisz and Harrison, 1971, p. 32). Edel (1972, p. 314), in fact, suggests that "both greenhouse industries and new career services could form part of the activities of a community development corporation or other ghetto development complex."

Another important concept of community develop-
ment strategies that cannot be detailed here, but should be mentioned, is integrated or collaborative businesses. Thus, certain industries would be set up to supply the needs of "guaranteed outlets" such as government agencies, or retail outlets would be established to provide that market.

Harrison (1972, pp. 186-193) also sees public employ-
ment programs as a necessary part of an overall strategy. His recommendation is based not only on the increasing need for public services and growth in the public sector, but also on the fact established in his research that for

minorities rates of return to education and training are far greater in the public sector than in the private. But these jobs must be genuine ones; not "leafraking" and not temporary.

Thus, the issues of the macro-performance of the economy and of its basic structure in terms of resource ownership and economic institutions come to the fore. In addition to micro-analysis, these have been the historic concerns of the discipline of economics. In particular, questions of income distribution and economic equity have moved to the top of the economic agenda as a result of the apparent failures of capitalist societies to solve their most pressing social problems. But analysis has its limitations; the achievement of full employment and economic equity depend ultimately on political organization and action. Hence, the success of New Careers and paraprofessional programs depends, in the final analysis, on the success of broader political movements.

## SUMMARY

The theoretical and research literature on the economics of paraprofessional employment presents myriad difficulties of evaluation. The most important questions concern models and goals. Is human capital theory or dual labor market theory the correct perspective from which to view paraprofessionalism? Should these choices of models change with the extent of employment — causing a change in the mode of evaluation as national employment levels change? To what extent should analysis extend beyond first order effects, beyond microeconomic analysis? To what extent should non-economic factors, the desirability of income redistribution and economic equity constitute elements in economic evaluation? What mix of public and private benefits should be present in a cost-benefit analysis? Finally, how do we develop complete and reliable data for control purposes, for cost estimation, and for value of benefits?

Economists have tended to divide themselves between two pursuits—those Sweezy has called "social science" and "social engineering" (1970, pp. 6-7). The former is an attempt to understand the totality of the economic system or some large part of it; the latter concerns itself with devising "ways and means of manipulating *given* institutions and variables to achieve results which for one reason or another are considered desirable." Unlike Sweezy, Solow believes that "little-thinking" is the most fruitful approach so long as it does not lead to "too single-minded a focus on how the parts of the machine work at the cost of a failure ever to ask whether the machine itself is pointed in the right direction" (1967, p. 101).

With respect to the evaluation of training and employment programs, "little-thinking" has perhaps properly dominated the field, but often, in Solow's words, it has degenerated "into mini-thinking or even into hardly thinking at all." By this, it is meant that the conventional cost-benefit studies have tended to limit the investigation to microeconomic variables and tended to ignore noneconomic variables altogether. At their best, such studies provide limited, albeit useful inputs to public policy; at their worst they can be misleading altogether. Perhaps the most serious shortcoming of this approach is the failure to place the observations and conclusions in a broad theoretical context concerning the operation of labor markets, and the economic system as a whole. For example, in the context of a stagnant and high unemployment rate, it is a reasonable conclusion that improved employment experience among trainees has its counterpart in worsened experience for others. To reach beyond primary effects is perhaps the most important contribution economists can make in the area of public policy; their ultimate concern is with the performance of the economic system in terms of its efficiency and in terms of the equity of its outcomes. If this judgment is true for tax, monetary, or tariff policy, it is equally true for manpower training and employment programs and paraprofessionalism as well.

## REFERENCE NOTES

1. Nixon, R. A. Luncheon remarks. *National Manpower Policy Task Force, Conference on Upgrading and New Careers,* Washington, D.C., 1970, 62-72.
2. Pointer, A. Y. *New professionals for public elementary schools: An analytical study of a college based manpower training program for Head Start follow-through staff.* Ph.D. Dissertation, Brandeis University, 1973.
3. Cleckley, B. J. *A study of new careers and upward mobility of new professionals in neighborhood health centers.* Ph.D. Dissertation, Brandeis University, 1974. 227 pages.
4. Walker, D. K. *Factors affecting the supply of labor in selected paramedical occupations in a local labor market.* Ph.D. Dissertation, University of California (Davis), 1975.

## REFERENCES

Barsby, S. L. *Cost benefit analysis and manpower programs.* Lexington, Mass.: D. C. Heath, 1972.

Berg, I. *Education and jobs; the great training robbery.* Boston; Beacon Press, 1971.

Brecher, C. *Upgrading blue collar and service workers.* Baltimore: Johns Hopkins University Press, 1972.

Brown, W. F. Effectiveness of paraprofessionals: The evidence. *Personnel and guidance journal,* 1974, *53,* 257-263.

Cohen, R. *"New careers" grows older.* Baltimore: Johns Hopkins University Press, 1976a.

Cohen, R. "New careers" a decade later. *New York University Educational Quarterly,* 1976b, *8,* 2-13.

Conant, E. H. *Teacher and paraprofessional work productivity. Lexington, Mass.: D. C. Heath, 1973.*

Doeringer, P. B., & Piore, M. J. *Internal labor markets and manpower analysis.* Lexington, Mass.: D. C. Heath, 1974.

Edel, M. Development vs. dispersal: Approaches to ghetto poverty. In M. Edel & J. Rothenberg (Eds.), *Readings in urban economics.* New York: Macmillan, 1972.

Gartner, A. *Paraprofessionals and their performance.* New York: Praeger, 1971.

Gartner, A., & Riessman, R. The paraprofessional movement in perspective. *Personnel and Guidance Journal,* 1974, *53,* 253-256.

Gartner, A., & Riessman, R. New careers. *New York University Education Quarterly,* 1977, *8,* letter to editor.

Grosser, C., Henry, W. E. & Kelly, J. G. "Prologue," pp. 1-11 in Grosser, Henry & Kelly (Eds.) *Nonprofessionals in the Human Services.* San Francisco: Jossey Bass, 1969.

Hamermesh, D. S. *Economic aspects of manpower training programs.* Lexington, Mass.; D. C. Heath, 1971.

Harrison, B. *Education, training, and the urban ghetto.* Baltimore: Johns Hopkins University Press, 1972.

Hoffman, A. M., & Warner, R. W. Paraprofessional effectiveness. *Personnel and Guidance Journal,* 1976, *54,* 494-497.

Matlack, L. R. Public service careers and new careers. In C. R. Perry, B. E. Anderson, R. L. Rowan, H. R. Northrup, et al. (Eds.), *The impact of government manpower programs.* Philadelphia: Industrial Research Unit, University of Pennsylvania, 1975.

New York Times, August 4, 1979 1,24.

Pearl, A. Paraprofessionals and social change. *Personnel and Guidance Journal,* 1974, *53,* 264-268.

Perry, C. R., Anderson, B. E., Rowan, R. L., Northrup, H. R., et al. *The impact of government manpower pro-*

*grams.* Philadelphia: Industrial Research Unit, University of Pennsylvania, 1975.

Rosen, S. M. Credentials—two strategies. In F. Riessman, S. M. Rosen, J. Featherstone & A. Gartner (Eds.), *Essays on new careers: social implications for adult educators.* Syracuse, N.Y.: Syracuse University Publications in Continuing Education, 1970.

Scheffler, R. M. Physician assistants: is there a return to training? *Industrial Relations,* 1975, *14,* 78-89.

Solow, R. M. The new industrial state or son of affluence. *Public Interest,* 1967, *9,* 100-108.

Sweezy, P. M. Toward a critique of economics. *Monthly Review,* 1970, *21,* 1-9.

Thurow, L. C. Secondary labor market effects of manpower programs: Comment. In M. E. Borus (Ed.), *Evaluating the impact of manpower programs.* Lexington, Mass.: D. C. Heath, 1972.

Thurow, L. C. Generating inequality. New York: Basic Books, 1975.

U. S. Bureau of Labor Statistics. *Monthly Labor Review,* 1975, *98,* 79.

U. S. Bureau of Labor Statistics. *Monthly Labor Review,* 1976, *99,* 91.

U. S. Bureau of Labor Statistics. *Employment and Earnings,* 1977, *24,* 43.

U. S. Bureau of Labor Statistics. *Employment and Earnings,* 1979, *26,* A-10.

U. S. Department of Health, Education and Welfare. *Overview study of employment of paraprofessionals.* Washington, D. C.: 1974.

Vietorisz, T., & Harrison, B. *The economic development of Harlem.* New York: Praeger, 1970.

Vietorisz, T., & Harrison, B. Ghetto development, community corporations, and public policy. *Review of Black Political Economy,* 1971, *2,* 28-43.

# New Careers: Where Have All the Flowers Gone?

Franklyn N. Arnhoff,
*Department of Sociology,*
*University of Virginia*

In a period of a little over a decade, the New Careers-paraprofessional movement has moved from a zenith of governmental and professional development and active promulgation to a nadir of inactivity and almost obscurity. In a recent extensive study of this movement and its programs, (Cohen, 1976) concludes that by 1975 "it was difficult to find any mention of 'new careers' programs or concepts in the human services literature" (p. 3). The Great Society programs and the War on Poverty that formed the larger panorama of which New Careers was but a motif, have also faded into the past. While not attempting a complete social history, an examination of

I appreciate the helpful comments and suggestions made on an earlier draft of the paper by Professors Gresham Sykes and Joel Telles.

some of the more pertinent factors involved in this rise and fall should be propaedeutic for the lessons of history: what happened and why.

Although the New Careers or paraprofessional movement came into vogue in the 1960s as part of a broader concern for social reconstruction and distributive justice, it has a far longer history, reflective of many divergent, yet intertwined themes. At the heart of these issues lie fundamental structural and functional relationships among the legitimating authority, class structure, and role of the service professions, all of which are intimately related to the division of labor. Ever since the first professional or higher skilled type decided to, or was encouraged to, divest himself of some segment of the duties and functions, that were thought undignified, burdensome, unappealing, or odious, new roles, functions, jobs, and job titles developed. New roles, of course, evolved spontaneously, while others emerged in response to some perceived need or want and were legitimized, frequently through conflict with existing authority. I am not suggesting that this is all that is and has been involved in the New Careers movement, but much of what has transpired under this general heading is an extension of broader developments in social structure and in the labor market, and represents the recrudescence of recurring themes in American social process. The term "human services" now encompasses a rather bewildering array of people, professions, agencies, occupations and functions, many of which are very recent, while others, such as the clergy, medicine, and law, date back to antiquity.

The groups that are aggregated under the comprehensive rubric of "human services," pose almost insurmountable problems for precise conceptualization and analysis. There is a tendency inherent in such grouping to suggest or imply a natural relatedness that transcends the very disparate societal subsystems involved. Each of these loosely articulated social subsystems such as health, education, welfare, criminal justice, mental health, often only articulate at the margins, if at all. Each, in its own right, has been repetitively criticized as constituting a non-system, the most egregious example being the health care system. Thus, the problems beg for analysis on the level of the overall social system rather than on the level of the putative successes or failures or the issues that may be unique to each or any of the paraprofessional groups.

Before progressing further, a brief digression is in order to deal with the term "paraprofessional" itself.[1] (No respectable paper on this topic can fail in its duty to address this matter.) The term is generally seen as a communication convenience for purposes of aggregation, and less pejorative than the often used synonyms of non-professional or subprofessional. The simple term "new, or allied _____ workers" (fill in the blank for the specific field) has been used but never really caught on. It is, important to note, since the mention of "legitimating authority" in the paragraph above alluded to power and control structures, that the term paraprofessional immediately sets a power and status relationship to a higher order which in this instance—the human service fields—tend to be predominantly the professions of medicine, law, social work, nursing, and education. The evolutionary history of each of these professions is quite different, yet each in its own way, and to a greater or lesser extent,

----

[1] Early difficulties with the definitional problem were noted well by Goldberg; "Various definitions of the unfortunate term *nonprofessional* are given. Here, it will be used to refer to persons who fail to meet the formal credentials for 'professional' positions in a given social agency. Thus, a person with a B.A. degree might be regarded as a nonprofessional in a highly professionalized family agency but as a professional in a department of public welfare . . . 'new nonprofessionals' are persons who are assuming a wider range of social welfare tasks, including, in some cases, direct service, than nonprofessionals have usually performed in the past. There are middle-class, new nonprofessionals as well as lower-class workers." Goldberg, G. S., Nonprofessionals in the human services, in C. Grosser et al. (Eds.), *Nonprofessionals in the human services*, San Francisco: Jossey-Bass, 1969, pp. 13-14.

came into being and was legitimized through prolonged struggles for autonomy, recognition, and power.[2] Ultimately, and in every instance, the final legitimacy is conferred by the state through certification and/or licensing, yet struggles for power, dominance, and control continue within, and between, these groups. Paraprofessionals exist only in relation to the parent professional groups whom they serve[3] despite heightened governmental activity to establish and/or hasten their legitimacy. The issue is of no small consequence for a later discussion of the aggregate human service fields.

Since the issues involved are so diverse and the vantage points for analysis and discussion encompass the broadest range of public policies, it will be helpful to briefly examine some manpower policies that are historically and conceptually pertinent.

## MANPOWER POLICIES

The term "manpower policies" is used to describe a wide range of governmental activities that are more or less, specifically addressed to the issues of unemployment, poverty, and inflation, and are part of a larger set of policies which have been described as "active labor market policies" (Ulman, 1974). For the most part, it has been an area in which analyses have been primarily the province of economists and political scientists. In the late

[2] See, for example, Hughes, E. C., *Men and their work*, New York: Free Press, 1958; Freidson, E., *Profession of medicine*, New York: Harper and Row, 1970; Berlant, J. L., *Profession and monopoly*, Berkeley: University of California Press, 1975; Krause, E., *Power and illness*, New York: Elsevier, 1977.

[3] They neither own nor control the means of production or service where they work; they function only in employee status; and most usually, even where certified or licensed, are specifically under the supervision of a professional or professional surrogate. The selective use or non-use of such personnel is also usually the decision of the controlling profession.

1960s, however, a wider range of social and behavioral scientists involved themselves in this area. While the Scheuer Amendments to the Economic Opportunity Act in 1966 are generally seen as the cornerstones of the New Careers movement, modern manpower policies have a considerably longer history.

> The Federal government began granting financial aid to the states for vocational education during the First World War (under the Smith-Hughes Act of 1917); it established what is now known as the Federal-State Employment Service and also an apprenticeship policy in the 1930s (under the Wagner-Peyser Act of 1933 and the Fitzgerald Act of 1937, respectively). However, it did not directly establish occupational training programs and subsidies until the early 1960s, with the passage of the Area Redevelopment Act in 1961, the Trade Expansion Act in 1962, and most important, the Manpower Development and Training Act (MDTA) that same year (Ulman, 1974 p. 87).

Add to this the vast range of legislation dealing with unemployment and poverty[4] and a temporal dimension of governmental manpower policies emerges to place the new careers movement as merely a very recent continuation rather than a unique phenomenon. What is in fact qualitatively different about the New Careers movement is, first, the attempt to accelerate the pace of change of job development and the division of labor, and second, to broaden the targeting of specific population segments as the beneficiaries of these changes.

All such manpower and economic policies ultimately deal with people and are addressed not only to the wealth of the society, but also to the utilization of people in pro-

---

[4]See, for example, Piven, F. F., & Cloward, R. A., *Regulating the poor,* New York: Vintage Books, 1971; Steiner, G. Y., *The state of welfare,* Washington, D.C.: The Brookings Institution, 1971.

ductive social roles, which in turn has considerable bearing upon the stability of the social order. However, a major trend became manifest in the late 1920s which continues to grow in importance: people have become a surplus commodity. Issues of population explosion aside, the reference is to the continued failure of the economy to provide employment to vast numbers of people in the traditional goods-producing sector of it with the resultant explosion of the service sector (Ginzberg, 1968). The response of government has to a very great extent mirrored its approach to other surplus commodities such as rice or wheat: subsidization of the producers, artificial price supports, and attempts to increase consumer demand. (The government has not attempted to introduce international export in this area, although transcending state boundaries [job mobility] is a matter of some concern.) This issue has not been introduced frivolously, but rather, as a legitimate similarity that serves to explicate the human, capital, labor, and professional issues against a background of a political and social belief system which is, at least to date, incapable of dealing with fundamental social realities. Consequently, neglect and exploitation unfortunately continue. Paraprofessionals in the human services cannot be evaluated or assessed independent of these social and economic policies since, in every instance, they are prodromal to the developments of the 1960s.

## THE DEVELOPMENT OF A SERVICE ECONOMY

To state that people have become a surplus commodity is not to negate human concerns, but merely to focus on a dimension that still occupies a prominent part of our social value system, as well as the psychological economy of most members of our society—the desire to be gainfully employed, engaged in productive work, and for the work to be meaningful, at least to the jobholder. It is of no small consequence that much of the rhetoric of the new careers movement was addressed not only to employment per se, but also to the proviso that the employment be personally satisfying, socially useful, and lead to a true career. If the late 1960s saw some lapses from the traditional Puritan ethic, at least on the part of some of the young, it was a momentary lapse, and work continues to provide not only the wherewithal for sustenance but an identity for most. But the nature of work or, at least the opportunities for the kind of work one does, have been continuously changing for about three decades.

The first and perhaps the most critical factor:

> Is that over the last three and a half decades advances in technology and other factors contributing to higher productivity enabled the goods-producing sector of the American economy to turn out a greatly enlarged output without any significant increase in employment. The important point to note is that it was not only a few industries which showed this trend, but the goods-producing sector as a whole (Ginzberg, 1968 p. 43).

Concomitantly, there has been: 1) continuous growth in the service sector (of which the so-called human services are a part); 2) a huge segment of which falls within the public and/or not-for-profit classifications; 3) a vastly different, markedly pluralistic economy which is in sharp contrast to the prevailing belief of an Adam Smith free enterprise system. Given this historical development, it is noteworthy that a good deal of what is involved departs markedly from concerns for survival and subsistence (needs) and relies upon "wants"—evolved, derived, inculcated, and manipulated,—but, nevertheless, involving things and services that are wanted. This service sector, which accounts for almost the total growth in post-World War II employment, "in 1974, accounted for two-thirds of total employment and $534 billion of output." (Ginzberg, 1976, p. 28)

## NEEDS, WANTS, AND DEMANDS

Regardless of the specific field or social problem under discussion, whether in professional journals or congressional testimony, the presentations always proceed on the basis of statements of what is needed, or at least, what is perceived to be needed to achieve a stated goal or end result. There is, however, an unfortunate tendency to interchange the terms "need," "want," and "demand" as if they were in fact synonymous. Although these are terms in common usage, they are used in manpower and economic analysis where there is promise of some greater clarity. There is no *single* definition of the term "need" in either manpower or economic usage and none that is universally accepted. We can, however, differentiate between two quite different usages. "Need" is often defined as whatever professional, scientific, or expert opinion considers necessary or required for desired ends. This type of use obviously differs considerably in its precision, depending to a very great extent on the degree and exactitude of knowledge and data in the particular expert's field; demonstrated cause-effect relationships, e.g., vitamin D is *needed* to prevent rickets, in contrast to assumed or reasonable relationships between, for example, poverty and the elimination of crime. Thus, it is useful to consider "need" as a matter of biological or social structural necessity, and "want" as a manifestation of psychological preference or desire. In common usage, and often in contrast to precise or expert opinion, is "need" meaning a desire for something, a want to be satisfied, a statement of social philosophy. Closely related is the derivative concept of "needy" as describing the poor, underprivileged, indigent ill, etc.

There is no question that a considerable portion of the

literature, both professional and popular, and the testimony of the "experts" that deal with needs in the human service areas, reflect the broad social philosophy and egalitarian concerns of many in our current society and culture. As Seeley wrote with regard to the mental health movement in 1953, and certainly others have observed, the entire concern for human services "is itself an expression of, and a result of, a revolution in social values" (Seeley, 1953 p. 15) that extended into the whole of contemporary society. To categorize professional expressions of need more precisely as statements of wants or desires is not to view them as less deserving of consideration or less worthy of social pursuit. It does, however, remove the aura of precision and exactitude (if not rectitude) and should permit for greater realization that there are other wants by other members of the polity regarding the same social conditions.

Given a highly pluralistic society, wants are diverse in nature, and putative needs, themselves, tend to be differentially perceived as a function of who is doing the needing. Professionals tend to perceive the society from a vantage point that is highly weighted with their substantive foci as well as professional desires and wants (usually expressed in terms of need). The politician's concept of need may well, and often does, include his perceptions of what his constituency does or does not want. Thus, even "the good life" and the "good society" are open to contentious discourse. Viewed from this perspective, given the nature of the social problems addressed by the legislation, social programs, and professional rhetoric during the '60s under the aegis of the "Great Society," it should be clear that "wants" were paramount, while "need" was often moot. We shall return to the issue of wants and needs again, but first, some consideration of another term that also creates problems —"demand."

Even in the professional literature "need" and "demand" are often used interchangeably; the two are further confused by the imperative nature of the word "demand" as it is commonly used. Much of the confusion and the difficulty can be ameliorated by the simple expedient of viewing "demand" as the reality principle of human services—"demand" is the economic expression of need, that is, it is the concept of need (or want) backed up by the dollars to pay. No matter how far back in our history one cares to go, in each and every instance of attention to poverty, health, welfare, education, crime, and unemployment, even when the fundamental ideological/political differences were or could be transcended, correctives foundered on the magnitude of the economics involved.

By the time the paraprofessional movement had reached its crest in the late 1960s, economic reassessments were in order and had begun, not only due to the costs of the Vietnam war, but also by virtue of a positively accelerating growth curve of public expenditures and a decline in the national economy. As we all know now, most of the federal programs that were the primary source of monies for a vast range of academic programs and correlated efforts that produced employment for New Careers began to deaccelerate, a trend that has, for the most part, continued to the present. Thus, the fundamental matter of the dollars to pay for the implementation of need or want increasingly set the limits of accomplishment.

Demand also can be and often is measured in terms of use: e.g., use of services or types of facilities. This is a useful method for some purposes although it is subject to Parkinsonian inflation—the more clinics, hospitals, patients, litigation, educational innovations, etc., the more the same are perceived as needed, since there is always the latent assumption that assumes/implies current use is the most efficient, parsimonious, economical, scientific, or professionally justifiable. This approach, however, still ignores the issue of who pays.

There is an additional approach to "demand" that is increasingly seen as a matter of some concern. After years of inflated rhetoric by politicians, governmental agencies, professionals, and the mass media, heightened expectations and unrealistic hopes have been created and public demands (in the imperative sense) frequently expressed. But in the light of more sober (and somber) reflection and reassessment, many of these demands are seen to be in conflict with what is known about alleviating the problems or conditions; no additional amount of manpower of any persuasion will provide the solution. This is increasingly, and most glaringly, the case in the health field as applicable to a host of health or health-related issues. We shall return to this theme again.

## Means and Ends: The Rhetoric and the Reality

The desire to change fundamental behavior patterns of individuals and institutions is imbedded in American history; the programs of the Great Society and the War on Poverty were merely the latest phases of these efforts. Liebman (1974), writing on this period observed:

> One strain in the national mood, the dominant strain at that moment, among the educated, professional, managerial classes was both that institutional arrangements could be imagined (indeed, could be selected by reason) which would produce whatever social circumstances were desired, and that technology had infinite capacity to produce the good life, at low cost. (p. 15)

What was desired (and promised) was an absolute increase in material well-being—the level of goods and services, housing, schools, hospitals and jobs; to alter the way people tended to think about themselves, their communities and their society, and to encourage greater participation in the political process by those traditionally underrepresented. Recognizing the economic underpinning of these social goals, economic policy received massive attention. Phelps (1974) described it as "one of the grandest experiments in social theory of this century," based upon an experiment "in high pressure macro-economic policy." (p. 32)[5]

What followed was a full panoply of governmental programs: poverty, housing, education, health, civil rights, urban redevelopment, and law and order. Paraprofessional New Careers jobs and programs were encouraged; they developed in all these areas. Each area spawned its own array of legislation and programs with its own subgoals, timetables, and production quotas. And each program, the nature of the federal political process being what it is, carried a specific mandate to articulate with and accommodate to the others. This was a fallacy, of course, but it had enough pressure behind it to dilute and diffuse efforts from the beginning, and to guarantee a mixed and spotty record. The usual statistics, produced for administrative and congressional purposes, dealt with the dollars spent, the number of programs funded, and the number of people *estimated* to be in training of various sorts and/or employed in their new roles.

During this same time frame, there was growing disenchantment with the social system—its failure to meet the needs of the people, its high costs, elitist orientation and domination, inequality and lack of equity, and so forth. The system, itself, became an object for change and many of the paraprofessional programs were viewed as vehicles for affecting fundamental changes in the functions, structures, operations, and organizations of American social, political, and economic institutions. This litany of change was common to all political persuasions—from the Marxist left to the reactionary right—change and destroy the

[5] This discussion merely served to demonstrate the ideologic climate at the time and its historical continuity. Any attempts to understand the developments of these programs at this time, certainly must seek other than ideology: Piven F. F. & Cloward, R. A. *Regulating the poor* (1971) present such a view emphasizing the changed labor market, migration patterns, and racial factors which were conducive to social unrest and the necessity for political intervention.

status quo, change the present to recapture the status quo, and resurrect the past. Goals, therefore, became not only multifaceted, but often contradictory, and the rhetoric of the social change agent provocateurs was heady indeed. The New Careerists themselves, often provided with the training and/or jobs to lift them out of poverty, were seen by their mentors and trainers as *the* agents of social change who, by their very presence in the existing institutions, would perform as Trojan horses, agitating from within to affect fundamental reform. Yet, when such workers, chosen for their indigenous qualities, began to enjoy upward mobility, changed their values and identified with their new socio-economic status, and moved out of the ghettos and slums, they were attacked by their mentors for their failure to keep the faith and to perform radical miracles. Since the purposes and motivations were so disparate, success on one dimension was often failure on another. If the Trojan horse idea, those lowest on the rung of prestige, money and power affecting major institutional changes seems preposterous, it was, nevertheless, a very seriously espoused goal.

But critique is not just a virtue of hindsight; there is hardly a point that can be presently made that was not voiced at the time by those within, as well as outside, of government; stated either as caveats to guide program development, or as warnings of the crash after the high, they were usually taken as the messages of Cassandra.[6]

In addition to the intent of providing jobs for the poor and accomplishing basic social reform, the paraprofessionals were to serve as additions to the professionals in areas of perceived personnel shortages. This substitution

[6]See, in particular, Grosser et al., *Nonprofessionals in the human services*, 1969, especially the chapter by G. Goldberg, pp. 12-39: Kurzman, P. A., *The new careers movement and social change: Social casework*, 1970, Jan., pp. 22-27: Pearl, A. & Riessman F., *New careers for the poor*, New York: Free Press, 1965; Arnhoff, F. N., Jenkins, J. & Speisman, J. *The new mental health workers*, in F. N. Arnhoff, E. A. Rubinstein, & J. Speisman (Eds.), *Manpower for mental health*, Chicago: Aldine, 1969.

of personnel is an economic commonplace and an accepted tool of manpower policy, particularly when it can reduce the cost of a given output. Given the accepted shortages of higher-priced professionals and the increasing awareness that it would never be possible to produce enough professionals to satisfy existing needs, lesser trained (cheaper) personnel doing the lesser skilled components of the professional's job, held the potential for freeing the professional and extending his skills, as it were, for high level, professional, skilled tasks.

The alleged shortage of professionals in all areas of the human services, especially in the health field, is intimately related to the social class of the service recipients. Although shortages across the social class spectrum were acknowledged, the deficiencies were most noteworthy for the poor and underprivileged with the various professions cited for their disinclination to provide them with services. The idea of the poor serving the poor, with its potential for rigidifying existing class differentials, while an issue of considerable debate, soul-searching and rationalization, nevertheless stands as a phenomenon of continued, rather than, diminished importance.

In essence, these three themes (jobs for the poor, extension of professionals for service delivery, and social reform) were the avowed, manifest goals of these programs. Needless to say, many proponents saw the priorities differentially; those who believed social reform was primary tended to view the provision of employment of the poor as a ploy to deaden the thrust of social activism. The issue of social reform, aided by growing opposition to the Vietnam war, grew in intensity until it often seemed to overshadow all other programmatic concerns. A more covert theme, the deflection of militancy and the assurance of social stability, became increasingly manifest as war dissatisfaction was more overt and socially disruptive, culminating in the "law and order" programs that also made use of the paraprofessional movement for its own ends.

It is the built-in paradox that American social values

from the beginning of the Republic espoused ideas of producing better citizens and a better society, yet implementing such ends must not be disruptive of current institutional and organizational power arrangements. The role of public policy, with regard to poverty and unemployment as a vehicle for the regulation of the poor and the abortion of social disruption, has been intensively studied by Piven and Cloward (1971). As their detailed exposition concluded, public welfare systems serve two main functions: the maintenance of civil order and the enforcement of work. Although one can disagree with whether these are main or secondary functions, they are, nevertheless, functions of some consequence. Our recent history bears testimony to the concerns for social order and the roles unemployment and inadequate compensation play in engendering social unrest. The utilization of national manpower policies to contain, mitigate and/or deflect militancy and civil disturbance are not necessarily conducive to problem management and solution in areas such as health, education, and the general delivery of human services. To the extent that such political considerations dominate substantive programs, one can expect exploitation of the program recipients and deflection of substantive goals. The latest expansion and contraction of programs and funds involving welfare and manpower policies has been amply demonstrated on the paraprofessional scene and is quite consistent with the fate of similar programs mounted in the past. Although multiple explanations are needed to account for these recent changes, certainly one factor has been the dramatic change in the perception of the degree of social disorder and the quality and quantity of overt militancy. It is particularly interesting to note that Pearl and Riessman, among other early writers in this area, were well aware of the potential for such exploitation of the paraprofessional; they saw the low-income indigenous paraprofessional as a latent "indigenous stool pigeon" serving the people he works for at the expense of the people with whom he lives since the intent of the employer was often to use the New Careerist to "cool" his neighbors (Pearl and Riessman, 1965, p. 196).

The varied programmatic motivations are obvious; less obvious, perhaps, are the implications of such political, rather than substantive, factors for career development, job stability, and meaningful social roles. I suspect but have no data to confirm my supposition, that those specific programs whose primary motive for inception was maintenance of community stability tend to be those that have disappeared, while those with more substantive task and service delivery underpinnings show a markedly higher survival rate.

Finally, for those for whom ideology provides the primary motivation in explaining the inception of these governmental programs, it is instructive to examine budgets to at least assess relative, if not absolute, commitments since " . . . a social program is usually better defined by its budget than by the language of the enabling legislation" (Ginzberg, 1974, p. 216). For the period 1965 to 1970, essentially the short life from the birth of these programs until their fall from grace, the areas of health, education, welfare, and housing—those areas most concerned with human services—were each funded by approximately $3 billion in new outlays (after deducting social security tax payments for Medicare). For perspective, remember that these program goals were aimed at fundamental reforms of chronic massive social problems; the budget of the Department of Defense, during the same period, increased from $46 billion to $77 billion (Ginzberg and Solow, 1974). By all criteria of magnitude of problem and commitment of resources, the human service programs were underfunded, lacking in broad-based congressional commitment, and projected on far too short a time scale—means hardly matched ends.

## Results and Assessments

Since the paraprofessional movement was part of a much grander effort at social reconstruction and economic policy development, evaluation of the outcome and results would be a mammoth undertaking far beyond the scope of this volume. Within the narrower focus of the New Careers, the differential area-by-area discussions in the rest of this volume is essential for in-depth analysis of specifics. Yet, there are aggregate views that do transcend the specific fields, and nagging questions that remain unanswered.

Despite the drastic decline in the human services literature as a whole, and a continued absence of definitive numbers and carefully controlled, hard data studies on impact, one conclusion is inescapable: area-by-area analysis reveals a variety of job titles and position classifications at the less-than-full professional level that did not exist a decade ago. It is certainly not possible to attribute all of these to this movement as many other factors were operating during this same period: it is still not possible to obtain consensus as to who should be considered paraprofessional. The difficulties involved in obtaining data were well summarized in a 1974 report by the Social and Rehabilitation Service.[7] In addition to the definitional problem they cite, data presented are frequently based upon those completing training rather than on those employed; on the federal level alone, the paraprofessional movement has been conducted under 100 different grant-in-aid programs authorized by 35 separate Congressional Acts and administered by eight departments and agencies. (Data for the states and municipalities involved would be even more staggering); since data collection is

[7] National Study of Social Welfare and Rehabilitation Workers, Work and Organizational Contexts. Overview study of employment of paraprofessionals (Research Report No. 3). Washington, D.C.: Social and Rehabilitation Service, DHEW, 1974. Quoted in Cohen, R., "New Careers" grows older, (1976, pp. 34-35.)

expensive, many agencies do not collect extensive statistics. If one were to simply total all the available estimates, disregarding the caveats mentioned above as Cohen (1976, p. 56) has done, then approximately 1.5 million people are employed as paraprofessionals. Approximately 250,000 of these are teachers' aides, and various traditional categories in the health field account for the majority of the rest. Even a recent, NIH-sponsored volume titled, *New Health Practitioners* was unable to determine precise or definitive data for the health field (Kane, 1975).[8]

If it is difficult to assess the net impact on the total labor market with any precision, it appears reasonable to conclude that regardless of specific causes, more people now occupy positions that are often classified as paraprofessional than was the case in 1965; representing the overall, if accelerated, continuation of the labor trends in the service sector described earlier. That is not much of a statement, but what is more important, given the focus of this movement on the poor and traditionally uneducated unemployables, is whether they have benefited by these programs to any significant extent. It is salutory to recall at this point that solving putative manpower shortages was also one of the goals of the time, and a marriage of convenience was arranged to help the poor, break the cycle of poverty, and so forth—employ the unemployables. As early as 1966, a study conducted for the Community Action Program (Yankelovich, 1966), based on projects in nine major cities, revealed that "creaming" was already a problem (hiring the most qualified, most capable, and most employable). Only 25% lacked a high

[8] In the health field in particular, the definitional problem looms large. Although physicians often tend to classify all non-medical types as paraprofessional (paramedical), there remains the question as to how much of the reported growth has been in paraprofessional jobs (those requiring minimal education) and how many in the ranks of the semi-professionals and technicians (physical therapists, inhalation therapists, etc.). All evidence seems to point to the latter as being primarily responsible.

school diploma, and 20% had some college education; hardly hard-core unemployed, yet an early demonstration of the dilemma of the mixed goals of eliminating poverty while providing the potential for quality service.

There are indications that this continues to be the case at the present time although labor market and employment opportunities have shown such drastic changes that assessment is even more difficult than before. Analysis of the Public Employment Program under the Emergency Employment Act of 1971, however (U.S. Government Printing Office, 1974, pp. 151-158), showed that only 18% were considered poor or disadvantaged, 14% were former welfare recipients, but almost 75% had at least a high school education. It is, of course, possible that various state and local data may show better batting averages in targeting on the chronic poor and unemployable, but there is little evidence for much optimism in view of overall labor trends. One can only reluctantly conclude that the helping of the poor aspect of the paraprofessional movement is not noteworthy for its success.

If realization of the goal of providing employment for the poor is at best conjectural, what benefits can be ascribed to these programs to date? Two facets to the question suggest themselves; demonstration of improved and more extensive service delivery, and a lesser considered benefit—that to the existing professions and institutions.

Over the years, from the earliest studies to the present,[9] there has been convincing evidence that people with less than full professional education, training, and credentials can, in fact, perform a variety of human services tasks including delivery of various kinds of direct services. The majority of such studies fall within the category of "program effectiveness studies"—the demonstration that "it is possible to accomplish the stated program or to implement a particular policy" (Arnhoff, 1975). Far

[9]See, for example, Grosser et al., *Nonprofessionals in the human services,* (1969); Cohen, R., *"New Careers" grows older,* (1976) for references and studies of evaluation and impact.

more difficult and contentious is the demonstration of "program benefits." Moreover, one of the most ephemeral and often nebulous facets of benefits is the question of quality. The health field, in particular, is probably the most glaring example of this problem, where even what constitutes quality medical care by the physician himself is an ongoing discourse of confusion. Successful demonstration of quality along dimensions of task specificity and definition offers promise, and where relevant, assessment according to the accepted technological base of the position. For those positions which are essentially the provision of advice, counseling, or other manifestations of a warm body and a sympathetic ear, however, evaluation of effectiveness, benefit, and quality fall heir to all the unresolved conceptual and methodological difficulties inherent in the evaluation of psychotherapy.

If there is question or uncertainty as to the primary effects of the paraprofessional movement in accomplishing some of its stated objectives, there would appear little difficulty in demonstrating the benefits for the professions and agencies involved. In 1967, Riessman, writing about paraprofessional training and employment, estimated that at least 50,000 training and supervisory personnel would probably be needed for employing 1 million nonprofessionals. The accuracy of the specific prediction aside, the period saw a rapid expansion of educational, training, governmental, and private contractor personnel; a multiplication of academic programs, program developers, managers, assessors and researchers; a developing business in films, cassettes, programmed learning texts, etc.; academic proliferation of books, monographs, papers, colloquia, training institutes, and endless meetings; countless millions poured into the colleges and universities for these activities; and a major thrust in the development of community colleges. While all this was of overall benefit to the economy and conducive to phenomenal growth for at least a few of the social science disciplines, it does point to an interesting matter of proportionate benefit. If the poor benefited only marginally, if existing labor market trends were merely accelerated, all the others involved, in the words of Tom Lehrer, did very well by doing good.[10]

From the beginning, the New Careers movement was an overly-romantic and rather naive overstatement of social hope for a small segment of a larger tableau that captured and captivated many social scientists at the expense of their critical faculties and evaluative expertise. As part of the larger scene, New Careers played its role in focusing attention on continued defects and deficiencies in our social structure. It is impossible to extract from the total zeitgeist what can be attributed to the paraprofessional movement per se; while the New Careerists hardly realized the dreams of being *the* agents of social change within the existing system, it would be equally amiss to dismiss their role as noncontributory to the developments of the time.

### Conclusions

If, as has been said, an army moves on its stomach, then a modern industrial society moves on its economy. But despite the esoteric theories and mathematical wizardry of modern economics, economists are unable to provide useful solutions to today's nagging social problems (Lekachman, 1976). Yet, the basic, if hoary, adage that "there is no such thing as a free lunch" can only be ignored at risk. The paraprofessional movement qua movement and its parent Great Society foundered in an economic morass that continues to bedevil not only this

[10]That what is dysfunctional for one purpose may be functional for another is not exactly new: consider the impact on the economy if all those involved in dealing with disease, poverty, crime, etc. were no longer needed due to miraculous cures of all these ills. There are some virtues for otherwise negatively valued social conditions. See, for example, Gans, H. J., The Positive functions of poverty. *American Journal of Sociology,* 1972, 78, 275.289.

country but all of western society. It is by looking at this scene that the current and future status, and ironies, of paraprofessionalism can be better understood.

For the past few years unemployment of considerable magnitude has been a rather invariate specter with underemployment a concomitant problem. Here, the individuals involved are not only the more or less traditional chronic poor and minorities, but also the middle-class, extending into the college educated; a phenomenon not seen in any magnitude since the great depression of the 1930s, and one that grows worse with each passing year. This part of the labor pool continues to silt-up with each graduating class that continues to pour out of the manpower pipeline. College enrollments (allowing for basic age-related population changes) continue to decline, college curricula have become increasingly skill- and occupation-oriented, and income differentials between high school and college graduates have shown a precipitous drop. The result has been overeducated and overtrained people occupying lower level, traditionally less educationally demanding jobs. Consequently, there are increasingly fewer opportunities and demands for those who have minimal or no formal education, a situation that conspires to decrease, not increase, the likelihood of opportunities for these target populations of the New Careers movement. What opportunities in this area exist are probably, for the most part, those that continue under the diminished governmental programs addressed to racial, sexual, and other minority imbalances.

The greatest growth in New Careers (both dollars spent and people employed) has been in the health and health related component of human services. The health industry, loosely defined, is now the nation's largest single industry with expenditures of more than $130 billion in 1976; it is also the nation's largest single industry employer with more than 4.5 million employees (Endicott, 1972). True, many of the jobs continue to be "de facto" handoffs from one group to another in a field notorious for professional rivalries, obsolete job structures, and misuse of human resources (HEW, 1971). Yet, the 422 health related job descriptions do continue to be a source of employment (Subcommittee on Consumer Economics of the Joint Economic Committee, 1973).

But after a decade of rising entitlements characterized by an explosive demand for human services, the translation of a variety of wants into needs and both wants and needs into human rights, ironies abound and are exemplified by the legal, educational, and health systems. In the legal field, for example, "paralegals," usually working under the supervision of a lawyer, execute many tasks previously performed by lawyers as well as some functions not previously provided or which were provided only in a limited way.[11] But a growing lawyer surplus, resulting in many newly admitted members of the bar failing to find employment, has stiffened resistance to the use of paralegals. Even more interestingly, there is increasing demand for reform of the legal system itself and attempts to *decrease* both the necessity for, and the involvement of, lawyers in many routine social affairs (e.g., elimination of lawyers for uncontested divorces, etc.).

In the field of public education, after years of using the educational system as a dumping ground and teachers as parent surrogates for a host of functions traditionally the task of the family, church, and other social institutions, teachers' aides have been growing in number, freeing the teachers (hopefully) to devote more time to teaching. But there is a horrendous glut of teachers, a back-to-basics teaching movement developing in reaction to national trends in decreasing accomplishment and achievement of the young, and school budgets cut in reaction to cost spi-

[11] *Paralegal personnel for attorneys general's offices,* Management Manual No. 6, National Association of Attorneys General Foundation, Raleigh, N.C., 1976; Statsky, W. P., The education of legal paraprofessionals: Myths, realities, and opportunities, *Vand. L. R.,* 1971, *24,* 1,083-1,084; *New careers in law: 2,* American Bar Association Special Committee on Legal Assistants, Conference Report, June, 1971.

rals. The educational system is increasingly called to task. Teachers' aides are among the "frills" that are being cut.

The entire health and health care delivery system is a matter of national debate and governmental investigation due to professional medical rigidities, soaring costs, and increasing realization that a progressively growing number of "health" demands and wants are beyond the scope of knowledge, or are not ameliorated by the intervention of health personnel or dollars since they reside in individual life styles and preferences and/or have their etiology elsewhere in the environment or social system. While health remains a markedly labor intensive field, this employment curve, too, shall not positively accelerate forever.

What is most ironic is that in each and every instance, all other factors notwithstanding, there is increasing public awareness that the failures to provide solutions (or, more realistically, effective management and containment) for social problems are the result, of defects in the system: the cosmetic changes that have characterized most past efforts are no longer sufficient. The rhetoric is rarely stridently radical now, and there is nothing that even approaches consensus as to what the defects are; yet even the most adamant establishment types[12] and Adam Smith[13] fundamentalists increasingly call for change in the "system." As to national comprehensive long range

[12] An excellent and interesting example is provided in a recent speech by Robert S. McNamara at an Annual Meeting of the World Bank; ". . . We must design an effective overall development strategy that can both accelerate economic growth and channel more of the benefits of that growth toward meeting the basic human needs of the absolute poor . . . the existing political order is in itself an obstacle to that growth." Quoted by Rosenfeld, S. F., *Washington Post*, September 30, 1977.
[13] Adam Smith, the classical political economist, favored free competition because it favored economic growth, but what is more often forgotten is that "he favored economic growth because only economic growth was likely to improve the condition of England's poor." Lekachman, R., (1976 p. 95).

health, education, and social policies and programs, G. B. Shaw's comment on Christianity is appropriate: "It is not that it has failed, it has never been tried."

REFERENCES

Arnhoff, F. N. Social consequences of policy towards mental illness, *Science,* June 2, 1975, *188,* 1277-1281.
Cohen, R. *New Careers grows older,* Baltimore: Johns Hopkins University Press, 1976, pp. 3; 56.
Dept. of Health, Education and Welfare. A White Paper, *Towards a comprehensive health policy for the 1970s,* Washington, D. C.: Government Printing Office, 1971.
Endicott, K. M. The Doctor dilemma. *Manpower,* July, 1972, 3.
Ginzberg, E. *Manpower agenda for America,* New York: McGraw Hill, 1968, 43.
Ginzberg, E. The pluralistic economy of the U.S., *Scientific American,* December, 1976, *234,* (6), 28.
Ginzberg, E. & Solow, R. M. Some lessons of the 1960s in E. Ginzberg, & R. M. Solow (Eds.), *The great society,* New York: Basic Books (Harper Torchbooks), 1974, 216.
Ginzberg, E. & Solow, R. M. Introduction In *The great society,* New York: Basic Books (Harper Torchbooks), 1974, p. 10.
Grosser, C. (ed.) *Nonprofessionals in the Human Services,* San Francisco: Jossey Bass, 1969.
Kane, R. L. (Ed.), *New health practitioners,* Washington, D.C.: DHEW Publication No. (NIH) 75-875, 1975.
Lekachman, R. *Economists at bay,* New York: McGraw Hill, 1976.
Liebman, L. Social Intervention in a Democracy, In E. Ginzberg and R. M. Solow (Eds.), *The great society,* New York: Basic Books (Harper Torchbooks), 1974, p. 15.

Pearl, A., & Riessman, F. *New Careers for the poor,* New York: Free Press, 1965.

Phelps, E. S. Economic policy and unemployment in the 1960s In E. Ginzberg & R. M. Solow (Eds.), *The great society,* New York: Basic Books (Harper Torchbooks), 1974, p. 32.

Piven, F. F. & Cloward, R. A. *Regulating the poor,* New York: Vintage Books, 1971.

Riessman, F. *Issues in training the nonprofessional,* New York: New York University, New Careers Development Center, 1967.

Seeley, J. R. Social values: The mental health movement and mental health, *Ann. American Academy Political Soc. Sci.,* 1953, *286,* 15.

Subcommittee on Consumer Economics of the Joint Economic Committee, Hearings, Medical policies and costs, 93rd Congress, 1st Session, May 16, 1973, p. 138.

Ulman, L. The uses and limits of manpower policy. In E. Ginzberg & R. M. Solow, (Eds.), *The great society,* New York: Basic Books (Harper Torchbooks), 1974, pp. 83; 87.

U.S. Government Printing Office, Manpower Report of the President, Washington, D. C. 1974, pp. 151-158.

Yankelovich, D. Inc. A Study of the Nonprofessional in the CAP. Unpublished manuscript New York, 1966.

# II. PARAPROFESSIONALS:
# THE STATE OF THE ART

# Paraprofessionals in Mental Health

Alan Gartner,
*The Graduate School and University Center
of the City University of New York*

Whatever else it is that justifies the utilization of para-professionals[1] in the delivery of mental health services—to offset the shortage of professionals, to be more cost efficient, to establish clear rapport with the community to be served, to provide employment for the unemployed—it is in the effectiveness of the services that they deliver

The original version of this paper was prepared for *Paraprofessionals in mental health; theory and practice.* Social Action Research Center.
[1] Many terms have been used for the non-credentialed worker: non-professional, subprofessional, new professional, paraprofessional, aide, auxiliary, allied worker, community professional, community worker, new careerists, etc. Recently, the term paraprofessional seems to be most widely accepted and is the one we shall use.

where a final assessment of their contribution must rest. To state this as a goal does not, of course, assure that data are available to allow an accurate and complete assessment. In fact, such is not the case. As with other areas of human services work, one cannot easily establish clear cause and effect relationships. One is not able to say that a particular set of paraprofessional behaviors *caused* a specific outcome. Unfortunately, there are not many studies of clinical or therapeutic effectiveness conducted under rigorous conditions with such procedures as control groups, etc. One analysis (Karlsruher, 1974) reports nine such studies, while another (Durlak, 1973) 14. These statements are, however, valid, to a greater or lesser degree, cut across the entire range of human services at all levels of personnel. Indeed, it may well be that paraprofessional programs in mental health have been better studied than have other interventions.

The bulk of the staff of mental health institutions have been paraprofessionals. These are what we have earlier called (Gartner and Riessman, 1971) the "old paraprofessional." This is the psychiatric aide, to use the most common title, working in a hospital setting, engaged in therapeutic work. A highly-significant, well-controlled experiment conducted by Ellsworth (1968) indicates that the old type of paraprofessional can play a powerful role in the improved treatment outcome for hospitalized male schizophrenics.

Beginning in the 1960s, the National Institute of Mental Health sponsored a series of paraprofessional programs. The first of these was Rioch's Mental Health Counselors program (1963). It was designed to provide low-cost psychotherapy and at the same time provide useful work for women with grown children; their success as a parent was seen as an essential job qualification. Evaluation of patient progress showed that none changed for the worse, 19% showed no change, 61% showed some change: 35% slight improvement, 20% moderate improvement and 6% marked improvement (Rioch, pp.;

683-685). Follow-up evaluation three years later, supported the earlier competence judgment (Magoon, Jolann, and Freeman, 1969).

Similar to the Mental Health Counselors program in terms of the background of the women trained as counselors, the Child Development Counselors program at the Washington D. C. Children's Hospital differed from Rioch's program in that the counselors worked with patients of a different class background (Eisdorfer and Jolann, 1969). A similar cross-class effort was involved in the Albert Einstein College of Medicine Mental Health Rehabilitation workers project that also used mature women (Davidoff, 1969). Similar to these are programs using college students as therapeutic agents, efforts that crossed both class and age lines (Beck, Kantor, and Geleneau, 1963; Buckey, Muench, and Sjoberg, 1970; Cowen, et al., 1966; Gruver, 1971; Holzberg, 1964; Kreitzer, 1969; Mitchell, 1966; Rappaport, Chinsky, and Cowen, 1971). There are now more than 500 such programs (Zax and Cowen, 1972), and one study reports that not only did college students help chronic patients significantly, but they were more effective than trained, experienced mental health professionals engaged in similar activities (Poser, 1966).

Both students and other paraprofessionals have been used to conduct behavior modification programs (Mira, 1970; Ryback and Staats, 1976; Staats, Minke and Butts, 1970); an evaluative study of one such program reports that improvement in the desired target behavior was achieved in 18 of the 21 cases, no change occurred in three cases, and no cases showed any children becoming worse (Suinn, 1974). And for more than 30 years, the U.S. Army has used paraprofessionals (titled Behavioral Science Specialists) to work in hospitals, correctional facilities, family assistance agencies, and drug and alcohol rehabilitation programs. At present, there are approximately 1,100 such individuals in 33 different types of jobs (Garber and O'Brien, 1977).

Carkhuff and Truax conducted a program at the Arkansas Rehabilitation Research and Training Center to identify those characteristics that make for more effective counseling, and the use of lay counselors. There are two major experiments of interest. The first compared the work of lay therapists, clinical psychology graduate students and experienced therapists. They concluded that: "The lay mental health counselors were able to provide a level of therapeutic conditions only slightly below that of the experienced therapists and considerably above that of graduate student trainees" (p. 12).

Earlier work of the Arkansas group had isolated three factors as critical to therapists' effect upon the client: communicating a high level of accurate empathy, non-possessive warmth, and genuineness toward the patients. There were no significant differences between the three groups of counselors as related to communicating accurate empathy or non-possessive warmth. On the third factor, communicating genuineness to the patient, the experienced therapists showed significantly higher performance.

Summarizing the effect on patients of the work of the lay therapists, Truax, the project director wrote: "Research evaluation indicated highly significant patient outcomes in *overall improvement, improvement in self-care, and self-concern, and improvement in emotional disturbance*" (p. 26). (Emphasis in the original.)

The second study conducted at the Arkansas Center addressed, more closely, the effect of paraprofessional counselors. Approximately 400 patients, with personality or behavior problems, some retarded and with speech and hearing defects, at the Hot Springs Rehabilitattion Center, were randomly assigned to three different groups: 1) experienced professional degree counselors, 2) experienced counselors assisted by an aide under maximum supervision, and 3) to aides (former secretaries with little if any college but 100 hours of training) working alone under supervision.

Performance under the three patterns of staffing were measured based upon client work quantity, client cooperativeness; client work attitude; quality of client work; client dependability; client ability to learn; and overall client progress. On all measures the best results were obtained by the aides working alone under the daily supervision of professional counselors. The professional counselors working alone had the second best results, while the counselors plus the aide had the poorest effects upon clients (Truax and Lister, 1970, p. 334). Carrying their conclusions beyond this project, the authors state:

> the findings presented here are consistent with a growing body of research which indicated that the effectiveness of counseling and psychotherapy, as measured by constructive changes in client functioning, is largely independent of the counsellor's level of training and theoretical orientation. (p. 334).

As mentioned earlier, two studies (Durlak, 1973; Karlsruher, 1974) surveyed the research findings on paraprofessionals. Based on more than 300 references over the past 10 years, Durlak (1973:301) reports that, "Only six reports were discovered that cited negative results with respect to the clinical effectiveness of paraprofessionals." Of the 14 studies Durlak identified that used various experimental procedures to compare directly the therapeutic effectiveness of nonprofessional and professional personnel, in 7 of the 14, "lay therapists had achieved significantly better therapeutic results than professionals: in the other 7 studies, results for the two groups were similar. *In no study have lay persons been found to be significantly inferior to professional workers.*" (Emphasis in the original p. 301).

In the 27 studies reviewed by Karlsruher (1974), only five compared the differential effectiveness of professionals and nonprofessionals as psychotherapeutic agents; in eight studies the control group received no treatment, while in the remainder there were no controls.[2] In the 13 studies of programs serving in-patient adults, the non-professionals were able to change the behavior of the patients in 12 of them. In 7 of the 8 studies where there was a control of an untreated group, there was "a significantly larger change in the behavior of the group treated by the nonprofessionals than in a no-treatment control group" (p. 65). Karlsruher reports that the changes in behavior in the controlled studies included measures of such indices as overt behavior (Appleby, 1963; Carkhuff and Truax, 1965; Verinis, 1970); results of psychological tests (Buckey, Muench, and Sjoberg, 1970; Holzberg, Knapp, and Turner, 1967; Rappaport, Chinsky, and Cowen, 1971); perceptual and motor tasks (Poser, 1966; Rappaport, Chinsky, and Cowen, 1971); and discharge rate (Carkhuff and Truax, 1965).

In 6 studies of out-patients and in 8 studies of adolescents and children reviewed by Karlsruher, various deficiencies of design lead him to conclude that it was not possible to draw conclusions about treatment outcome.

## COMMUNITY MENTAL HEALTH PROGRAMS

Although some of the programs we have described have served out-patients, most were for hospitalized patients. Now we want to turn to programs which have their base in the community, including those which are a part of community mental health centers, as well as other programs that carry out similar activites.

The broadest examination of the work of paraprofessionals in mental health is Sobey's 1976 study of more than 10,000 paraprofessionals in 185 NIMH-sponsored

[2]Unfortunately, the studies reviewed by Durlak and Karlsruher differ and, therefore, their reviews are not strictly comparable.

programs. The major finding relates to the reason for the use of paraprofessionals.

> Nonprofessionals are utilized not simply because professional manpower is unavailable but rather to provide new services in innovative ways. Nonprofessionals are providing such therapeutic functions as individual counseling, activity group therapy, milieu therapy; they are doing case finding; they are playing screening roles of a non-clerical nature; they are helping people to adjust to community life; they are providing special skills such as tutoring; they are promoting client self-help through involving clients in helping others having similar problems. (p. 6)

The basis for the use of paraprofessionals is illustrated by the responses of project directors to the question of if, given a choice of hiring professionals, project directors would prefer to utilize paraprofessionals for those functions that professionals had previously performed. In short, 54% preferred to use paraprofessionals over professionals for tasks previously performed by professionals. The paraprofessionals performed three major functions: therapeutic, special skill training, and community adjustment; and five lesser ones: case finding, orientation to services, screening, caretaking, and community improvement. In 69 projects, the directors reported expanding the professionals understanding of the client group through association with the paraprofessionals (p. 161).

In summary Sobey found,

> Nonprofessionals were viewed as contributing to mental health in two unique ways: 1) *filling new roles based on patient needs* which were previously unfilled by any staff; and 2) performing parts of tasks previously performed by professionals, but tailoring

the task to the nonprofessionals' unique and special
abilities. (p. 174) (Emphasis added to quote.)

Perhaps because of the breadth of her study, Sobey
does not provide empirical data as to effectiveness vis-á-
vis consumers. Unfortunately, most of the studies of indigenous paraprofessionals suffer from a similar absence.

A 1969 survey of 80 community mental health centers
found that 42% of all full-time positions were filled by
indigenous workers. The figures were higher in drug
abuse treatment (60%) and geriatric service (70%) (National Institute for New Careers, 1970, pp. 14-15). A study
in the same year of paraprofessionals in 10 community
mental health centers in New York City reported their
"actual work as described by administrators varied from
unskilled to highly skilled but more often is of the highly
skilled variety" (Gottesfeld, 1970 p. 288). The work included interviewing, escort service, home visits, staffing
storefront offices, receiving complaints, collecting information, acting as translators, performing individual and
group counseling, organizing community meetings, leading therapy groups, assisting patients in self-care, acting
as patients' advocates with other agencies, casefinding,
screening applicants, making case conference presentations, doing casework, giving speeches, planning aftercare services, and giving supportive psychotherapy to
ex-patients.

The Lincoln Hospital Mental Health Services program
in New York City established three neighborhood centers, each staffed with between 5 and 10 aides. They were
seen as "bridges" between the professionals and community. They are expediters, advocates, and counselors.
Something of the power of their impact and the need for
services in a community such as the South Bronx is
shown by the service figure of 6,500 persons seen at two
of the centers in the first nine months. As the program
offered services to the clients' whole family, it was es-

timated that more than 25,000 persons were effected during that period (Riessman and Hallowitz, 1965).

Harlem Hospital in New York City has employed indigenous workers in a variety of roles. Harlem residents interested in working with the aged, provided outpatient geriatric psychiatric services. They made home visits, provided escort services, observed and reported on patient behavior, and provided social services. About half of the study group of 60 cases were successfully managed. Especially innovative was the Harlem Hospital Group Therapy Program, which used indigenous aides (Christmas, 1966). The aides worked in a half-day treatment program for a small group of chronic psychotic post-hospital patients. The aides participated as co-therapists in weekly group psychotherapy sessions, acted as participants and expediters in the monthly medication group meetings, were members of the weekly therapeutic community meetings, and lead the weekly client discussion groups. In addition, they performed case and family services, home interviews, surveyed patient needs, and provided community mental health education (p. 413). The program was expected to hold one-third of the patients; it held two-thirds (Wade, 1969 p. 678).

The Temple University Community Mental Health Center Philadelphia, Pennsylvania has trained indigenous workers as mental health assistants, workers whom they describe as "helpers first, then therapists" (Lynch, et al., 1968, p. 428). Over an extended period of time, a work pattern developed where the mental health assistants "function as a 'primary therapist' providing on-going treatment and continuity of care that would include the procurement of ancillary (professional) services whenever appropriate." (p. 429) The assistants, a title the workers themselves preferred to "aides," worked with 96% of the patients in the clinic's first year. Two key factors in their work involved "holding" patients and by their availability, preventing hospitalization.

The Central City Community Mental Health Center in Los Angeles used community workers in a program designed to develop additional mental health personnel, train new workers, improve understanding between the disadvantaged and mental health personnel, and increase the available services and create new services appropriate to the disadvantaged. The community workers were used in the mental health facility itself; at a family service center, in various social welfare agencies, in a public health project, in a public housing program, and to provide crisis intervention therapy in a suicide prevention program (National Institute for New Careers, 1970 p. 14).

In summing up his survey of nonprofessionals in mental health, Cowen, (1973) states, "Collectively, non-professionals are doing virtually everything that professionals do; they are also involved in new activities not heretofore considered part of MH (mental health) services" (p. 448).

## When Paraprofessionals Are not Effective

Given their widespread utilization, one has to consider the issue of effectiveness. Effectiveness involves both a question of purpose and comparison. Durlak (1973) reports that based upon a survey of more than 300 studies, "only six reports were discovered that cited negative results with respect to the clinical effectiveness of non-professionals" (p. 301). Karlsruher (1974) reports that of eight studies involving controls, seven "reported a significantly larger change in the behavior of the group treated by the nonprofessionals than in a no-treatment control group" (p. 65); in the eighth study, there was an equal amount of change in the treated and untreated groups.

It is fair to conclude, as Albrecht (1973) states, "If the major goal of the indigenous nonprofessional is solely to render effective therapy and service, then the movement seems able to meet this goal" (p. 247). Within the context of this goal, however, there are factors that mitigate successful performance and tend to make the activities of paraprofessionals ineffective. These include "excessive dependency, panicking, projecting one's problems onto others, lack of sophistication." (Cowen, p. 448). Beyond the particularities of work behavior, there are the broader issues of contradictory demands. Elsewhere, Gartner, (1970) said that the paraprofessional is expected to be "worker and consumer, force for change and member of the system, critic of professionalism and aspirant professional" (p. 61). Thus, there is role ambiguity (Halpern, 1969) that involves the question of whether the paraprofessional is to be a "bridge" from the community to the profession (Christmas, Wallace, and Edwards, 1970), or do the professions' menial tasks, or bring services to the unserved and new services to others; in other words, what are the underlying conceptual bases (Arnhoff, Rubenstein, Speisman, 1969) for new mental health personnel?

As Minuchin (1969) points out, "The inclusion of paraprofessionals in the existing structure of delivery of services brought to a head the bipolarity of approaches to mental illness which was already incipient in the field." (p. 724) Although some see the paraprofessional efforts as co-optive (Haug and Sussman, 1969) or pacification (Statman, 1970), or "an ill-conceived and unrealistic effort" (Ritzer, 1973 p. 227), Minuchin argues that the paraprofessional must be both force for, and product of, a reconceptualization of the very relationship of individual and society.

The future of paraprofessionals will be considered in a separate chapter in this volume. It seems appropriate to note, however, that it is not only that paraprofessionals are a significant percentage of the present mental health work force which give importance to assessing their effectiveness, it is also that they are the work force of the future.

REFERENCES

Albrecht, G. L. The indigenous mental health worker: The cureall for what ailment? In P. M. Roman & H. M. Trice (Eds.), *The Sociology of Psychotherapy,* New York: Jason Aronson, 1973.

Appleby, L. Evaluation of treatment methods for chronic schizophrenics. *Archives of General Psychiatry,* 1963, *8,* 476-481.

Arnhoff, F. N., Rubenstein, E. A., & Spiesman, J. C. (Eds.) *Manpower for Mental Health.* Chicago: Aldine, 1969.

Beck, J. C., Kantor, D., & Geleneau, V. A. Follow-up of chronic psychotic patients "treated" by college case-aide volunteers. *American Journal of Psychiatry,* 1963, *120,* 269-271.

Buckey, H. M., Muench, G. A., & Sjoberg, B. M. Effects of a college student visitation program on a group of chronic schizophrenics. *Journal of Abnormal Psychology,* 1970, *75,* 242-244.

Carkhuff, R. R. & Truax, C. B. Lay mental health counseling: The effects of lay group counseling. *Journal of Counseling Psychology,* 1965, *29,* 426-431.

Christmas, J. J. Group methods in teaching and action: Nonprofessional mental health personnel in a deprived community. *American Journal of Orthopsychiatry,* 1966, *36,* 410-419.

Christmas, J. J., Wallace, M., & Edwards, J. New careers and new mental health services: Fantasy or future? *American Journal of Psychiatry,* 1970, *126,* 1480-1486.

Cowen, E. L. Social and community interventions. In P. H. Mussen, & M. R. Rosenzweig, (Eds.), *Annual Review of Psychology,* Palo Alto, Calif.; Annual Reviews, Inc., 1973, *24,* 423-472.

Cowen, E. L., Zax, M. & Laird, J. D. A college student volunteer program in the elementary school setting. *Community Mental Health Journal,* 1966, *2,* 319-328.

Davidoff, I. F. The mental health rehabilitation worker: A member of the psychiatric team. *Community Mental Health Journal,* 1969, *5,* 46-54.

Durlak, J. A. Myths concerning the nonprofessional therapist. *Professional Psychology,* 1973, *4,* 300-304.

Eisendorfer, C., & Jolann, S. E. Principles for training "new professionals" in mental health. *Community Mental Health Journal,* 1969, *5,* 352-359.

Ellsworth, R. B. *Nonprofessionals in psychiatric rehabilitation.* New York: Appleton-Century-Crofts, 1968.

Garber, D. L., & O'Brien, D. E. Operationalization of theory in the training of paraprofessionals. *Journal of Education for Social Work,* 1977, *13,* 60-67.

Gartner, A. Organizing paraprofessionals. *Social Policy,* 1976, *1,* 60-61.

Gartner, A., & Riessman, F. The performance of paraprofessionals in the mental health field. In G. Caplan (Ed.), *The American Handbook of Psychiatry.* New York: Basic Books, 1971.

Gottesfeld, H. A study of the role of paraprofessional in community mental health. *Community Mental Health Journal,*1970, *6,* 286-290.

Gruver, G. G. College students as therapeutic agents. *Psychological Bulletin,* 1971, *76,* 111-128.

Halpern, W. I. The community mental health aide. *Mental Hygiene,* 1969, *53,* 78-83.

Haug, M. R., and Sussman, M. B. Professional autonomy and the revolt of the client. *Social Problems,* 1969, *17,* 153-161.

Holzberg, J. D. Chronic patients and a college companion program. *Mental Hospitals,* 1964, *15,* 152-158.

Holzberg, J. D., Knapp, R. H. & Turner, J. L. College students as companions to the mentally ill. In E. L. Cowen, E. A. Gardner, & M. Zax (Eds.), *Emergent approaches to mental health problems.* New York: Appleton-Century Crofts, 1967.

Karlsruher, A. E. The nonprofessional as a psychotherapeutic agent: A review of the empirical evidence pertaining to his effectiveness. *American Journal of Community Psychology,* 1974, *2,* 61-77.

Kreitzer, S. F. The therapeutic use of student volunteers. In B. F. Guerney, Jr. (Ed.), *Psychotherapeutic agents: New roles for nonprofessionals, parents, and teachers.* New York; Holt Rinehart and Winston, 1969.

Lynch, M., Gardner, E. A., & Felzer, S. B. The role of indigenous personnel as clinical therapist. *Archives of General Psychiatry,* 1968, *19,* 428-434.

Magoon, T. M., Jolann, S. E., & Freeman, R. W. *Mental health counselors at work.* New York: Pergamon, 1969.

Minuchin, S. The paraprofessional and the use of confrontation in the mental health field. *American Journal of Orthopsychiatry,* 1969, *39,* 722-729.

Mira, M. Results of behavior-modification program for parents and teachers. *Behavior Research and Therapy,* 1970, *8,* 309-312.

Mitchell, W. E. Amicatherapy: Theoretical perspectives and an example of practice. *Community Mental Health Journal,* 1966, *2,* 307-314.

National Institute for New Careers. *New careers in mental health: A status report.* Washington, D. C.: University Research Corp., 1970.

Poser, E. G. The effect of therapist training on group therapeutic outcome. *Journal of Consulting Psychology,* 1966, *30,* 283-289.

Rappaport, J., Chinsky, J. M., & Cowen, E. L. Innovations in helping chronic patients. *College students in a mental institution.* New York: Academic Press, 1971.

Riessman, F., & Hallowitz, E. Neighborhood service centers program: A report to the U.S. Office of Economic Opportunity on the South Bronx neighborhood service center, December, 1965.

Rioch, M. National Institute of Mental Health pilot study in training mental health counselors. *American Journal of Orthopsychiatry,* 1963, *33,* 678-698.

Ritzer, G. Indigenous nonprofessionals in community mental health. In P. M. Roman & H. M. Trice, *The Sociology of psychotherapy.* New York: Jason Aronson, 1973.

Ryback, D., & Staats, A. Parents as behavior therapy-technicians in treating reading deficits (dyslexia). *Journal of Behavior Therapy and Experimental Psychiatry,* 1970, *1,* 109-120.

Sobey, F. *The Nonprofessional revolution in mental health.* New York: Columbia University Press, 1970.

Staats, A., Minke, K., & Butts, P. A token-reinforcement remedial reading program administered by black therapy-technicians to problem black children. *Behavior Therapy,* 1970, *1,* 331-353.

Statman, J. Community mental health: The evolution of a concept in social policy. *Community Mental Health Journal,* 1970, *3,* 5-12.

Suinn, R. Training undergraduate students as community behavior modification consultants. *Journal of Counseling Psychology,* 1974, *21,* 71-77.

Truax, C. B. *An approach toward training for the aide therapist: Research and implications.* Fayetteville, Ark. Arkansas Rehabilitation Research and Training Center, 1965.

Truax, C. B., & Lister, J. L. Effectiveness of counselors and counselor aides. *Journal of Consulting Psychology,* 1970, *17,* 331-334.

Verinis, J. S. Therapeutic effectiveness of untrained volunteers with chronic patients. *Journal of Consulting Psychology,* 1970, *34,* 152-155.

Wade, R. The view of the professional. *American Journal of Orthopsychiatry,* 1969, *34,* 676-680.

Zax, M., & Cowen, E. *Abnormal psychology: Changing conceptions.* New York: Holt, Rinehart, and Winston, 1972.

REFERENCE NOTES

1. Fishman, J., & Mitchell, L. New careers for the disadvantaged. A paper presented to the annual meeting of the American Psychiatric Association, May 13, 1970, San Francisco, Calif.

# Paraprofessionals in Health-Care Delivery: An Overview

Betty Jane Cleckley,
*School of Social Work,*
*University of Tennessee*

In the last decade, the health care system has witnessed an upsurge in the participation of paraprofessionals in the delivery of services. This effort developed primarily as a result of increased public attention, interest, and concern devoted to the enormous problems existing in the health-care system: organization and availability of health-care services; inequities in care; rising costs; duplication of costly services; maldistribution of manpower; shortages of personnel; and problems of utilization (Califano, 1977). Moreover, problems of unemployment, underemployment, and poverty generally contributed to the employment of paraprofessionals (U.S. Department of Health, Education, and Welfare, 1974).

This chapter will review factors that contribute to the utilization of paraprofessionals and describe the experiences of this new kind of personnel in the health-care delivery system. While the context in which paraprofessionals are examined is primarily neighborhood health care centers and New Careers, the chapter also describes the experience of paraprofessionals in other types of health settings such as hospital outpatient departments, clinics, and public health facilities.

In health-care delivery to the poor, the focus of change has centered on more direct community involvement. The stated concern of the federal government for community involvement was described by the former Secretary of Health, Education and Welfare, John Gardner (1969):

> Institutions should be designed to strengthen and nourish each person . . . which will not just serve the individual but give him an opportunity to serve. When people are serving, life is no longer meaningless, they no longer feel rootless. (pp. 40-41)

Such concern has led to changes in public policy, expressed in the passage of enabling legislation, and government support of programs such as Neighborhood Health Centers and New Careers. Since these two are the most visible of the programs designed to increase the number of paraprofessionals in health-care delivery, they will constitute the focus of this discussion.

## NEIGHBORHOOD COMPREHENSIVE HEALTH CENTERS

Neighborhood Comprehensive Health Centers, established by the Economic Opportunity Act of 1964, led to the development of a new health-care structure designed to operate in the interest of the patients rather than in the interest of the providers of care. Three basic components were incorporated in the creation of these centers. The primary concern was to provide comprehensive, dignified, high-quality ambulatory care to poor people for the maintenance of health and the treatment of illness. An additional component was consumer participation. By serving on neighborhood health councils, advisory boards, or health associations, community residents would gain valuable experience in planning and decision-making. Finally, these centers would provide opportunities for training and employment at both the professional and paraprofessional level (U.S. Congress, 1964; 1966).

Three such projects were undertaken initially: Tufts Community Health Action Program in Columbia Point, Boston; Gouverneur Ambulatory Center—Beth Israel Hospital, New York City; and the Department of Health and Hospital Center, Denver (Abrams, 1971).

The concept of the neighborhood health center is not new in America. Aspects of the program and some of the functions of this innovation appeared early in the 19th Century in the ambulatory-care programs of dispensaries and public health departments (Jonas and Rimer, 1977).

The inception of Neighborhood Comprehensive Health Centers, however, introduced an important innovation—the utilization of paraprofessional workers in the delivery of health care. Staffing these neighborhood centers focuses on the employment of poor, disadvantaged, and minority-group members, and the provision of training and education to enable these new employees to move into the higher paying job market. By offering these enlarged job opportunities for community residents and providing suitable training and education, Neighborhood Health Centers were responding to the health agencies component of the New Careers program as established by the Scheuer-Nelson Amendment (U.S. Congress, 1966).

## NEW CAREERS

Paralleling the development of Neighborhood Health Centers, the New Careers program has been an equally-important effort that influenced the utilization of para-professionals in health-care delivery. This legislation represents another attempt to make the health-care system more responsive and effective in meeting the needs of the poor.

The legislation mandated that programs both in public and private agencies should be designed to improve the physical, social, economic, or cultural conditions of the community in various fields such as health, education, and welfare. Among other important objectives, the Amendment stipulates that programs must be designed to, "assist in developing entry-level employment opportunities in human services, provide maximum prospects for advancement and continued employment without federal assistance, and be combined as necessary with education, training, and counseling, transportation assistance, and such other supportive services as may be needed to assure the entry into full-time and permanent employment as careers" (U.S. Congress, 1966, p. 749). In other words, a specific aim of New Careers is to provide funds for employment, education, training of the poor, and to make it possible for low-income persons to be promoted to higher positions.

Similar goals are included in the 1967 and 1969 amendments to the Economic Opportunity Act of 1964, and in the 1973 Comprehensive Employment and Training Programs (see U.S. Code, 1975). It is noted that 112 New Careers projects were in operation in the human services fields as of June 30, 1969 (U.S. Department of Labor, 1970). According to Gartner (1973), more than a fifth of the slots of these programs were in health settings. In the House and Labor Reports on the 1967 Amendments, the intention of the legislation is clearly stated (Nixon, Note 1).

Primary emphasis is upon training which will lead upward on a career ladder. The first step would be work under (1) professional supervision at an entry level job with supplementary education, including basic education if necessary and enrollment in courses. The second step would be the (2) performance of work assignments requiring greater skill, emphasizing on-the-job training. The third step would be (3) a permanent position on an agency staff, with certification as necessary, such as for a practical nurse, an occupational therapist, an assistant teacher, a patrolman, and other civil service positions. (p. 7)

Clearly, the Scheuer-Nelson Amendment, with its provisions for New Careers and upgrading in accordance with the career ladder concept, represents an effort on the part of the federal government to resocialize the poor. Moreover, it seems that the federal government advocates a definition of manpower that stresses the development of human resources by helping disadvantaged individuals adapt to work situations and fulfill their work potential.

New Careers requires jobs offer the poor some measure of status, satisfaction, pride, and self-respect. The fact that the jobs should be permanent, allow for upward mobility, and have a place on a career ladder would indicate that New Careers is not just an ancillary program for the temporary utilization of large numbers of the poor. New Careers represents an attempt to achieve change in the health-care system.[1]

## REVIEW OF THE LITERATURE

A survey of the literature concerning the experiences

---

[1]See the article by Pearl elsewhere in this volume for a discussion of New Careers (Editor's Note).

of paraprofessionals involved in health-care delivery shows a predominance of studies about neighborhood health centers, particularly in relation to the extent to which they improve the quality of health care provided for the poor (see, for example, Savitz and Mauss, 1977; Office of Economic Opportunity, 1970; and Abrams, 1971). There is, however, a paucity of studies, either descriptive or evaluative, about New Careers in neighborhood health centers. There is almost no research on the extent to which paraprofessionals have maximized constructive utilization of health-care services by economically disadvantaged people. The few studies extant indicated that New Careers programs have concentrated on providing employment for poor residents. They show that some opportunities have been provided for low-income people to receive training and education as components of their work experience.

In Sparer and Johnson's (1971) evaluation of 33 OEO-funded neighborhood health centers, they found that approximately 6,000 paraprofessionals had been hired, constituting close to 50% of all staff employed in the centers. The evaluation also indicated the high interest of community residents in these positions. Practically all the centers had developed training programs. Some of the variables examined in training and utilization of paraprofessional staff that were the basis for rating the projects were: 1) whether priority was given to community people in selecting paraprofessional staff; 2) the degree of utilization of paraprofessionals in innovative roles; and 3) the adequacy of the training provided to paraprofessional personnel.

All of the centers were judged to have developed adequate training programs with respect to providing core curriculum and on-the-job training. Core curriculum refers to the formal presentation of information and skills relevant to paraprofessionals. A total of 19 out of the 27 projects employing paraprofessionals in service capacities tended to utilize them for housekeeping tasks and activities. Thus, paraprofessionals served in positions comparable to homemaker roles. In eight projects paraprofessionals assumed parts of the task previously performed by professionals. They worked, for example, as family health workers and provided functions generally assigned to public health nurses, social workers, and health educators. Sparer and Johnson (1971) considered the latter eight projects more innovative than the 19 projects that employed paraprofessionals as homemakers. In the remainder of the projects, paraprofessionals provided outreach services.

Zahn (1968) reported that the Montefiore-Morrisania Hospital demonstration project in New York City (currently Dr. Martin Luther King Health Center) was able to recruit residents from the poorest strata of the community to provide comprehensive health services, such as preventive, diagnostic, and follow-up. Of particular interest is her finding that, of the 109 paraprofessionals recruited, 85 remained in the program, receiving primarily on-the-job training and core curriculum. The latter was provided during an eight-week period to enable paraprofessionals to develop an understanding of health-care services and community resources. Further, paraprofessionals were informed of the existing and planned health careers. Through on-the-job training, paraprofessionals were trained as laboratory technicians, medical record assistants, home health aides, and the like. The center failed, in its effort to gain college credit for the core curriculum and on-the-job training provided to paraprofessionals according to Zahn (1968) because a satisfactory plan could not be worked out with colleges in the area.

The studies by Goldstein and Horowitz (1973) of the manpower situation, including manpower utilization, at 20 Boston area hospitals reinforces these findings. Studying 96% of 204 paramedical personnel at the hospitals, functioning as registered nurses, licensed practical nurses, nurse's aides, orderlies, and neighborhood health workers, the authors found that nurse's aides and orderlies constituted the lowest group in the nursing occupational hierarchy. Moreover, because of educational requirements and credentials, there was little, if any, opportunity for these workers to advance. Goldstein and Horowitz (1973) report that most of the workers said they would like to move up if they could.

Further evidence of this deficiency is revealed in another study in the Boston area, "New Careers and Upward Mobility of New Professionals in Neighborhood Health Centers" (Cleckley, Note 2). The data were gathered in three neighborhood health centers and the Boston Family Planning Program. The universe of paraprofessionals included those employed for both a long as well as a short time. Each agency employed between 150 and 160 paraprofessionals. Only 144 paraprofessionals, however, participated in the study. More than 94% of the participants were female. The low representation of men might have arisen from their attitudes toward these kinds of jobs as "women's work." Second, the low pay may have been a deterrent. Third, the lack of male participants may possibly be indicative of recruitment practices of these agencies (see Navarro, 1975).

The age distribution ranged from 19 to 64 years with a mean age of 32.8 years. Almost 25% of the respondents were under 25 years of age, 50% were 25-38, and 25% were 39 years of age and older. This pattern suggests that agencies were willing to employ young, inexperienced workers. Almost 62% of the participants were black; almost 15% were from other minority groups, including Puerto Ricans, other Spanish-speaking residents, and blacks from Haiti.

A total of 36% of the paraprofessionals either had some college education or were college graduates. Another 32% were high school graduates. Additionally, more than 75% of these participants were employed prior to accepting a job at the neighborhood health centers. These data indicate that a high degree of selectivity operated in the selection of area residents for employment.

The study found that new professionals employed in these centers had a variety of job titles such as medical assistant, community health worker, social work assistant, dental assistant, and family planning community educator. At the same time, the nature of the paraprofessionals' services and activities were accentuated by their ability to establish relationships and to communicate with other people and with professionals within the health center.

What is the upward mobility of new professionals? The study shows that, of the 114 participants in the subsample, 67 advanced primarily through salary increments and increased job responsibility. The result of the study also indicates that participants who achieved upward mobility were mostly black, married women between the ages of 25 and 38, with at least some high school education. Generally, they earned under $500 a month.

With respect to the types of education and training provided, for the most part, centers concentrated on providing on-the-job training and in-service training to a majority (44%) of the participants. Slightly less than 25% of the new professionals, however, received special technical training and college level courses. Nevertheless, the overall training pattern would seem to place limitations on mobility and career advancement of participants, because this type of training appears to be of most value to the specific center in which the paraprofessionals are employed. It is doubtful that such training would have a great deal of transferability to other centers or to other occupational settings (see discussion in Jonas, 1977: Chapter 4).

A follow-up telephone interview was conducted in 1978 to determine what had happened in these agencies with respect to education and training, job retention, and the development of career ladders. While unable to obtain specific statistics, the author discovered that the Boston Family Planning Agency had closed down. An administrator in one of the other centers reported that some

152 PARAPROFESSIONALS IN THE HUMAN SERVICES

paraprofessionals are still employed in entry level positions. There are no career ladders in existence or opportunities for career advancement, however, for these workers. Furthermore, she noted the agency has "undergone changes" that she attributes to the lack of federal support and interest in the paraprofessionals. Attempting to resolve the financial problems, they were in the process of developing a proposal designed to attract additional federal funds. According to the respondent it is hoped that paraprofessionals will be licensed to provide home health care.

Certain characteristics of paraprofessionals contribute to their being effective in health-care delivery. Among characteristics cited by Warnecke et al. (1976) in their study of 80 paraprofessionals working as health guides in a Central Buffalo project are: knowledge of the neighborhood, being of a similar social and cultural background as the residents served, having an activist orientation,[2] and an employment history prior to becoming a paraprofessional.

Critical support for the employment of paraprofessionals can be gained from another recent study. Wingert et al. (1975) sought to assess the effect that a year of "comprehensive health supervision would have on the health and welfare of indigent patients" and to "compare the effectiveness of professional public health nurses with that of health aides providing such health care supervision" in a pediatric outpatient department. The authors conclude that, of the seven paraprofessionals recruited from the community served by the hospital, five clearly demonstrated that they could be trained to carry out a complex system of tasks, make meaningful and responsible decisions regarding patients' health concerns, and contribute in each of these respective areas in a manner similar to professionals. There were, to some extent, differences between the professional public health nurses,

[2]See the Riley, et al., article elsewhere in this volume (Editor's Note).

with whom the paraprofessionals were compared, and the indigenous workers in their ability to identify specific kinds of problems such as visual and hearing impairments (Wingert, et al.). Paraprofessionals surpassed the professionals, for example, in making referrals to specialty clinics and helping patients to follow through with their appointments. On the basis of the findings, however, Wingert, et al. ascertained that there was no evidence "that any changes in the health and welfare of the study population occurred because of improved communication at a collegial level or because of common cultural interest" (p. 850).

In a comparable study that sought to document the impact of the introduction of a new class of paraprofessionals—family health workers—into a neighborhood health center, Fliegel (Note 3) judged that the project failed. These paraprofessionals, however, were introduced into a highly-politicized environment where the professionals saw their roles as ancillary and minimal while their trainers saw them as agents of change. This lack of consensus precluded any meaningful introduction of a new role, so the paraprofessionals became redefined as nurses' assistants and social work assistants. In these traditional roles, the paraprofessionals presented no threat to the professionals and were precluded from developing any innovative role.

An illustration of the effectiveness of paraprofessionals can be seen in the work of the Indian Health Service's effort to promote health among Indians and Alaskan natives (U.S. Department of Health, Education and Welfare, 1972). Paraprofessionals were employed from the community and from different tribal groups to provide services to their community. Working on the assumption that education and training are important to these community health representatives, the Indian Service established career opportunities and provided college and on-the-job training as well. As a result, the paraprofessionals have, for example, an opportunity to become social work associates, practical nurses, and dental assistants.

F. Daniel Cantrell, president of the National Association of Neighborhood Health Centers, points out that the peak development for neighborhood health centers was 1974. At that time, there were 200 neighborhood health centers throughout the United States. By 1977, however, only 25% of these centers were still in existance. He and Jonas both indicate that in the mid 1970s many health programs begun in the mid 1960s were cut back or dissolved for lack of adequate federal support (Cantrell, 1974; Jonas, 1977). Cantrell contends that there has been " . . . a wholesale abandonment of federal philosophies and practices which centers felt necessary for the effective delivery of health care to their patient population" (p. 60). Thus, the decline in the government support of neighborhood health centers has caused much concern; it is felt that this situation will decrease substantially the number of paraprofessionals in health-care delivery.

Although views vary concerning the cause of the problem, it is generally believed that the federal government never provided the adequate support to solidify the programs permanently within the health-care system. Stressing the facts that government often moves slowly and along traditional lines and usually with influential interest group support, Somers and Somers (1977) suggest that it would be difficult for innovations such as neighborhood health centers to gain the support of influential interest groups. Thus, their future may look dim at times.

Some writers, such as Breyer (1977), believe that while the theoretical idea of neighborhood health centers was promising, the centers have not worked well in reality. In a recent New Jersey study, Breyer found that the centers performed poorly in implementing effectively the objectives of neighborhood health centers. Observing that the centers failed to employ paraprofessional and new professional personnel, Breyer concluded that this situation hampered physicians and, as one consequence, the community was not provided adequate services.

## SUMMARY AND CONCLUSIONS

The literature suggests that paraprofessionals are used in a variety of ways in the health-care delivery system. In terms of paraprofessional manpower generated by Neighborhood Health Centers and New Careers, the effect has clearly been increased additions to the cadre of personnel. Further, there is considerable evidence about the value and effectiveness of the poor in providing health services. While the value of introducing paraprofessionals has been recognized, there is hardly any procedure or mechanism for integrating these programs into the mainstream of health-care delivery. Additionally, only to a limited extent have paraprofessionals been provided the kinds of education and training experiences they need for the development and achievement of a marketable skill.

New Careers in neighborhood health centers proposes a single solution for multiple social problems: service delivery, poverty, and manpower shortages. Upon implementing programs, administrators and developers have effectively placed poor people in service roles in the health-care system. It is partly through this method that neighborhood health centers are carrying out their responsibility to improve the quality and quantity of health services delivered to individuals and families in low-income urban and rural areas, and thus meeting a need vitally important to alleviating the problems of the poor. As a result, the New Careers concept of jobs first, with training and education built in, has been realized for some paraprofessionals.

And yet, true upward mobility for paraprofessionals in neighborhood health centers and in other health settings is severely restricted and generally remains a basic problem. An editorial in the *American Journal of Public Health* (Lynch, 1972) poignantly describes the situation:

> Despite the escalating utilization of new professionals (paraprofessionals) in health, we remain essentially second class citizens in the health manpower hierarchy, impacted at the bottom and out of the mainstream of the American health care system. Our roles are largely experimental in nature and are determined by others. The much talked about career ladders, where they exist, are low-level ladders, that do not pierce the credentials barrier. Training remains largely a function of the individual agencies in which we work, is not standardized within regional areas nor nationally and, thus, prevents job mobility. This lack of standardization also prevents meaningful credentials for our positions. (p. 623)

The absence of standardized job titles is an important barrier to job mobility for paraprofessionals in health delivery. The nature of the problem is discussed by Hicks (1972). She observes; "A job that formerly did not exist, that of family health workers, how has some 30 different names in about 200 programs across the country" (p. 30). Commenting on the obstacles to mobility, Hicks notes that a problem arises when a health worker seeks to change jobs within the field because of the variety of training programs, lack of standardization, and the fact that some of the training that new professionals have been provided is too specialized.

Barr (1967) writing about Mobilization for Youth 10 years earlier warned of this danger:

> And in the long range, there is the problem of economic segregation. In hiring large numbers of indigenous nonprofessionals, we may run the risk of creating a new group for whom upgrading is impossible—a group whose members will find themselves

"locked in" in the same sense that hospital attendants are prevented from moving up in the medical
world. (p. 17)

Thus, locking people into low-paying, dead-end service
jobs continues to be a festering problem in the health-care
system. Furthermore, perhaps as long as the career ladder concept is central to New Careers, the program will
continue to obtain minimal results. The history of the
program has shown that the career ladder approach has
not worked for a substantial number of persons. Persons
locked into low-paying, dead-end service jobs in the
health-care system are beginning to realize, moreover,
that there are avenues to upgrading other than the career ladder route; therefore, unionization is among the
possibilities gaining recognition and acceptance.

One of the major obstacles to the career ladder approach and to upward mobility within the health-care
system is the medical model that reinforces both unequal
status and differential power within the system. The
medical model and its hierarchical element contributes
to health professionals' controlling and influencing
health manpower, planning, and policy. The rigid controls of certification and licensure, restructuring the jobs
and utilization of paraprofessionals, attest to this situation.

It is unlikely that the current approach to restructuring jobs and tasks (the transfer of routine and menial
functions to less-trained personnel) will reduce the manpower shortage, lead to upward mobility, or alleviate poverty. Rather, it accelerates the process, already in
existence, whereby lower socioeconomic groups are ce-
mented into lower-status positions in the "secondary"
labor market.

According to Gartner (Note 4) what has occurred, in
effect, in neighborhood health centers "is the encapsula-
tion of the paraprofessionals at the bottom to serve angry,
critical, poor clients, who hitherto were not well served"

(p. 11). Gartner further states: "Even where neighborhood health centers are operated by or as part of hospitals, there is little articulation between the two systems, no doubt, in part at least, an expression of the limited articulation between the two service systems" (p. 11).

It appears that because paraprofessionals are hired to work solely with the poor in their communities, class barriers are reinforced and the poor are further locked into their communities. Rather than creating a situation where the poor are trained and employed to work with the poor, it might be more desirable to open up opportunities for low-income persons to live and work in the larger society, to move into the "mainstream" of American life.[3]

## IMPLICATIONS FOR THE FUTURE

In sum, the important skill of paraprofessionals in neighborhood health centers and in other settings, such as outpatient clinics and public health facilities, appears to be their ability to persuade community residents to continue to accept a parallel system of health care and services. The phenomenon reported earlier with respect to the dissolving of neighborhood health centers, however, would seriously impact the services paraprofessionals are providing. Closing the neighborhood health centers would decrease the number of jobs available and would have a profound effect on paraprofessionals' personal and family situations.

Assuming that prepaid group medical practice—such as Health Maintenance Organizations (HMOs)—will be the preferred type of health care in the future, it is important to consider the roles and responsibilities that paraprofessionals will have in this new delivery system. For example, are there provisions for outreach health work-

[3] A different perspective is shown by Arnhoff elsewhere in this volume.

ers? It would appear that HMOs as currently conceived lead to the employment of a different cadre of health practitioners, such as physician assistants, associates and nurse practitioners (Roemer and Shonick, 1973). Is it foreseeable that paraprofessionals could be trained in these disciplines, and such positions viewed as goals of upward mobility for them? Further, is it conceivable that HMOs, as developed by affluent and powerful interest groups in the private sector, will utilize paraprofessionals and be responsive to meeting equitably the needs of all persons? If HMOs are to serve as an important structure in reducing health care costs, then those who are trained as paraprofessionals should be able to extend their roles into this new system of care. Therefore, consideration of upward mobility should enter into the manpower planning process.

Whatever the future health care system or mechanism of payment (National Health Insurance), the achievement of upward mobility for paraprofessionals will continue to be a pressing and increasing problem. When the problems of education, training, and upgrading of paraprofessionals in the health-care system are considered, the concern of social policy should be directed first toward reforms within the public educational system and, second, toward the overall problem of getting the poor, many of whom are racial and ethnic minorities, admitted to technical and professional schools. To date, it is clear that advancement to higher paying primary jobs in health care delivery depends mainly upon technical and professional training and credentials that presently can be obtained only through formal education. In this way, it is hoped that the health-care delivery system will make provisions for recruitment, education, and training in institutions of higher education and develop career ladders with real potential for upward and lateral mobility among paraprofessionals, thus significantly improving their life chances.

REFERENCE NOTES

1. Nixon, R. A. *Legislative dimensions of the new careers programs: 1970.* Mimeographed. New York.
2. Cleckley, B. J. *A study of new careers and upward mobility of new professionals in neighborhood health centers.* Ph.D. Dissertation, Florence Heller Graduate School for Advanced Studies in Social Welfare, Brandeis University, 1974.
3. Fliegel, B. S. *Careers that failed: A case study of family health workers in a community health action system.* Ph.D. Dissertation, Florence Heller Graduate School for Advanced Studies in Social Welfare, Brandeis University, 1974.
4. Gartner, A. *Health systems and new careers.* Mimeographed. New York University.

REFERENCES

Abrams, H. K. Neighborhood health centers. *American Journal of Public Health,* 1971, *61,* 2236-2239.

Barr, S. A professional takes a second look. *The American Child,* 1967, *49* (1), 14-16.

Breyer, P. R. Neighborhood health centers: An assessment. *American Journal of Public Health,* 1977, *67,* 179-181.

Califano, J. A., Jr. National health care planning. *Vital Speeches,* 1977, *49,* 113-114.

Cantrell, F. D. Neighborhood health centers: A search for stability. *Urban Health,* 1974, *3,* 60-66.

Gardner, J. Toward a self-renewing society. *Time,* April 11, 1969, pp. 40-41.

Gartner, A. The impact of new careers on the American health system: An examination of its past, present, and future. *Career Development,* 1973, *2*(2), 2-8.

Goldstein, H. M., & Horowitz, M. A. Restructuring paramedical occupations. *Manpower,* 1973, *5,* 2-7.

Hicks, N. Health workers facing uncertainty with rapid expansion of training programs. *The New York Times,* March 19, 1972, p. 30.

Jonas, S. chap. 4. In *Health care delivery in the United States.* New York: Springer, 1977.

Jonas, S., & Rimer, B. Ambulatory care. In *Health care delivery in the United States.* New York: Springer, 1977.

Lynch, W., Jr. What new professional health workers want. Editorials. *American Journal of Public Health,* 1972, *62*(5), 623-624.

Navarro, V. Women in health care. *The New England Journal of Medicine.* 1975, *292,* 398-402.

Office of Economic Opportunity. *Healthright programs— the neighborhood health center.* (OEO Pamphlet 6128-9). Washington, D.C.: U.S. Government Printing Office.

Roemer, M. I., & Shonick, W. HMO performance: The recent evidence. *The Milbank Memorial Fund Quarterly: Health and Society,* 1973, *51,* 271-317.

Savitz, D., & Mauss, E. M. A community health project in 10-year perspective. *Public Health Reports,* 1977, *29,* 570-581.

Somers, H. M., & Somers, A. *Health and health care: Policies in perspective.* Germantown, Md.: Aspen System Co., 1977.

Sparer, G., & Johnson, J. Evaluation of OEO neighborhood health centers. *American Journal of Public Health,* 1971, *61,* 931-942.

U.S. Code. Work and training activities. In *U.S. Code 1970 edition, supplement V.* Washington, D.C.: U.S. Government Printing Office, 1975, 2455-2457.

U.S. Congress. *Economic opportunity act, 1964.* Section 222. Washington, D.C.: U.S. Government Printing Office, 1964.

U.S. Congress. Community action-adult work and employment programs. In *Economic opportunity act amendments of 1966.* Public Law 89:749, Section

206. Washington, D.C.: U.S. Government Printing Office, 1966.

U.S. Department of Health, Education and Welfare. *The Indian health program of the U.S. Public Health Service.* Health Services and Mental Health Administration. Washington, D.C.: U.S. Government Printing Office, 1972, 1-31.

U.S. Department of Health, Education and Welfare. Overview study of employment of paraprofessionals. (Research Report No. 3, Social and Rehabilitation Services UE-05417). Washington, D.C.: U.S. Government Printing Office, 1974.

U.S. Department of Labor. *National assessment of the new careers program: July, 1967—October, 1969.* Division of Public Career Programs and Training and Employment Service, Manpower Administration. Washington, D.C.: U.S. Government Printing Office, 1970.

Warnecke, R. B., Mosher, W., Graham, S., & Montgomery, E. B. Health guides as influentials in Central Buffalo. *Journal of Health and Social Behavior,* 1976, *17,* 22-34.

Wingert, W. A., Grubbs, J., Lenoski, E. F., & Friedman, D. B. Effectiveness and efficiency of indigenous health aides in a pediatric outpatient department. *American Journal of Public Health,* 1975, *65*(8), 849-856.

Zahn, S. Neighborhood medical care demonstration training programs. *The Milbank Memorial Fund Quarterly,* Part I, 1968, *46,* 309-321.

# Paraprofessionals in Education: A "Status" Report

Jeanne K. Wagenfeld,
*Jenkins Vocational Rehabilitation Center*
*Kalamazoo, Michigan*

This chapter will deal with the use of paraprofessionals in education. The traditional school system is comprised of professionals operating in three components and performing different roles and functions. It is necessary to specify briefly how the various professionals perceive their mission in order to understand the way paraprofessionals are used in each component. Further, as much of the literature indicates, the amount of consensus about the role and function of teachers, counselors, and administrators within the educational system and in society, in general, appears to be an important variable in understanding the relationship between professionals and their use of paraprofessionals.

Also briefly described here will be the history and legislation that made the use of paraprofessionals in the school a reality. The role of, and function of, each of the three levels of professional within the educational system will then be delineated and followed by a discussion of how, for each professional type, paraprofessionals were trained, used and evaluated.

## HISTORICAL PERSPECTIVE

It is generally agreed that a major impetus for the use of paraprofessionals in recent years came from the work of Pearl and Reissman. In their *New Careers for the Poor* (1965), they argued that paraprofessional employment in the human services could improve the delivery of these services and also provide a meaningful career ladder for those trapped in poverty. This idea, however, can be traced back at least several hundred years. The Elizabethan Poor Laws, enacted in England in the sixteenth century, stipulated that those people who failed to find gainful employment and who were consequently dependent on the state be trained to do "community improvement." Although this work was generally menial, the principle of training the unemployed to perform a public service was explicit in the provision (Bowman and Klopf, 1967).

In 1953, the Ford Foundation provided funding for an experimental program in Bay City, Michigan using auxiliary personnel in education. This program differed from the Elizabethan Poor Laws, the depression era Works Project Administration and the National Youth Administration in that the purpose was to increase the effectiveness of teachers by assigning the nonprofessional function to auxiliary personnel rather than providing work opportunities for the unemployed.

This program was negatively received by teachers who felt that the available educational funds should be spent on employing more teachers rather than on untrained personnel. Two similar projects funded by Ford Foundation followed: one in Fairfield, Conn. and the other in Rutgers, N. J., but there was no major break-through in the paraprofessionals in education in the late 1950s and early 1960s (Ford, 1961).

The major impetus for the use of paraprofessionals in education came in the mid 1960s with the passage of Title I of the Elementary and Secondary Education Act of 1965 (ESEA). This legislation was novel because it was the first time that federal money had been appropriated for public schools. The momentum for Title I was a perceived urgency to upgrade education in disadvantaged areas. The funding under Title I was available for direct payment to teachers and to advance instruction as part of an anti-poverty policy. As part of this legislation, $75 million was appropriated for teacher aides who would be employed in elementary and secondary schools in low income areas. There were, however, no criteria for employment selection or any implicit message that the poor should be recruited to work in their neighborhood schools (Bennett and Falk, 1970).

The second important thrust for paraprofessionals in education came with the Subprofessional Career Act often referred to as the Scheuer Amendment of the Economic Opportunity Act. This legislation appropriated $40 million in 1966-67 to be administered through the Department of Labor for the demonstration and training programs in New Careers for the poor. The Scheuer program provided nearly $89 million for the training and hiring of low income persons for career positions in public services (Title II, 1966; Title IB, 1967). In 1970 Public Services Careers incorporated the New Careers program into its program.

The main criticism of this program was that there was a narrowness in the selection of those unemployed persons who were chosen as New Career interns (Bennett and Falk, 1970). The basic criteria used for inclusion in the program were proper background interests and education. This limited the type of person employed considerably, and, in many ways, was counter to a comprehensive program to provide new careers for the poor.

A more comprehensive piece of legislation, as far as paraprofessionals were concerned, was the Education Professions Development Act (EPDA) of 1967. EPDA authorized a comprehensive training program in the human services areas. A total of $240 million was appropriated. It stated its main purpose as " . . . to test the hypothesis that the schools of this country can combine on *equal terms* with the colleges and universities to create viable programs for training teachers of teachers, whether these latter are experienced school personnel, graduate students, or teacher aides" (Announcement and Prospectus, 1968).

In 1969, emerging from the EPDA, the Career Opportunities Program (COP) was formed to address the following educational issues:

> strengthening the self and group identity of the children of the poor, minorities and alienated;
> using training programs as an instrument of, and catalyst for, educational change;
> bringing new and different persons into the school to play new and different roles; and
> developing relations of equality (parity) among participants, school communities being served, and colleges (Carter, 1977, p. 183).

COP became a national career training program that had three main goals. The first was to enhance the education of children of low income families by using educational auxiliaries who came from the same sociocultural milieu and who, it was believed, would inject some "relevance" into the schools. It was maintained that community residents would facilitate the educational services that teachers and administrators provided since their personal experiences would enable them to relate more empathically and effectively to the needs of low income children than could the middle class professionals. The second goal was to provide these paraprofessionals with opportunities to work their way through a career lattice where there was the possibility of vertical, horizontal, and diagonal mobility within the myriad of educational career opportunities. The third goal was to have some commitment from the state departments of education to modify state teacher certification requirements to include credit for experience gained through COP (COP, 1970).

As a result of this legislation, the entire field of education found itself in a situation of change. In the 1965-66 school year began 40% of all teacher aide programs (National Education Association, 1967). With the great increase in the number of paraprofessionals in education, there was considerable confusion as to how they could be utilized. Not surprisingly, the introduction of this new element in the school system created some perceived threats to the security of the professional staff. As will be seen in the following sections, the amount of role clarity and status that teachers, counselors, and administrators had about their own positions was an important desideratum of how defensively they felt and consequently, how they used, evaluated, and responded to paraprofessionals.

## Paraprofessionals in Teaching

*The Role of the Teacher.* In educational circles, as well as in society in general, a rather clearly defined role is that of teacher. Although the role of teacher is far more complex than is often seen by outsiders, there is general agreement about what a teacher does and who can use the title "teacher."

Kehas (1970) asserts that teachers are the only professionals who are fully accepted in education. The reason for this is based on how he perceives the basic structure of education. These structures are based on the following premises: 1) education is teaching; 2) the major objective of education is the teaching-learning function; and 3) the primary relationship in schools, consequently, is that between teacher and student. In a similar manner, Moser and Sprinthall (1971) view the schools as having defined their role as transmitters of academic ideas and having been primarily committed to intellectual development. Lucien (1952) states that the most widely recognized role of the teacher consists of the ability to plan, initiate, and evaluate the learning process. The amount of consensus about their role and function offers the teacher a certain amount of security.

Further protection is provided teachers by the fact that teachers have sole right to the title "teacher" as a result of certification. Certification is by state law granting the right of a person to be considered a member of the profession on the basis of meeting specified criteria. In the case of teachers, a Bachelor's degree with specified courses and experience is required in all 50 states and the District of Columbia. The implication of this is that, in order to protect the public, only those persons who are certified teachers can legally be involved in the act of teaching.

The security of this protection made the introduction of paraprofessionals in the form of teacher aides somewhat less threatening than in other sectors of education. The introduction of EPDA, however, gave rise to a movement headed by Don Davies, Director of EPDA, and others (Allen, 1970; Ryan, 1970; Sharpes, 1970) to view this as an opportunity to change the role of the teacher and make it more of a combination of instruction, coordination, and supervision (Denemark, 1974). It appeared, however, that although there were likely to be changes in the role of teacher with the introduction of large numbers of teacher aides, their status as teachers would not be threatened because they were certified.

*Teacher Aides.*   Although there has been tremendous increase in the number of teacher aides (250,000 people worked in this capacity in 1974), DeLaVergne and Blitz (1975) have noted that there still exists great confusion and lack of consensus about their appropriate function. Problems regarding the role and function of the aides were reported in 23 states and centered on what constituted teaching and nonteaching functions (Tanner and Tanner, 1969).

If one looks at the ways paraprofessionals have been used in teaching, they fall into three categories: technical, supportive, and supplementary (Bennett and Falk, 1970). Those activities that are subsumed under the "technical" category really run the gamut from collecting lunch money, doing routine record keeping, helping to prepare and assemble materials, to running audiovisual equipment. If a state has defined teaching in a narrow way, however, then covering a study hall would not be permitted since a student may ask a question which would call for professional judgment (Tanner and Tanner, 1969).

The "supportive" role requires the aide to undertake supportive educational functions under the supervision of a teacher. The aide in this capacity would be involved in individual tutoring and supervision of reading groups. In Minneapolis, the teacher's role is so defined so that he/she can assign the paraprofessional an instructional task (Bennett and Falk, 1970). Here, again, how teaching and nonteaching was defined in the state made a difference in what the aide was permitted to do. Finally, the "supplementary" function involves enriching classroom activities by sharing one's unique talents and experiences.

Although the activities that paraprofessionals could conceivably perform are specified by these three categories, this approach has resulted in great chaos and confusion. Nearly half of the states have reported difficulty discriminating between teaching and non-teaching functions. In order to remedy the situation, some efforts have been made to create a continuum between professional and non-professional activities and a different use of staffing patterns in the schools (Tanner and Tanner, 1969).

In its handbook on the use of auxiliary personnel in the schools, the U.S. Office of Education articulated guidelines that specified those tasks they viewed as being in the professional domain (Carter and Dapper, 1972). Those pertaining to teaching were: diagnosis of student needs, prescribing instruction programs, selecting appropriate materials, presenting or teaching content, and evaluating student progress.

The handbook states that the auxiliary personnel do only those things requested by the teacher and under his/her direct supervision. The teacher's discretion, however, is allowed. "Depending on his/her skill, ability, training and interest, the school volunteer may be called upon to perform more complex tasks related to the reinforcement of instruction" (p. 16).

In order to further clarify their functions, Anderson (1966) proposed three categories of aides: the non-professional, the pre-professional, and the paraprofessional. The non-professional aides are those who do not want to become teachers, have no college training, and serve in the role of an assistant. This would require little or no formal training and whatever training was required would be on-the-job. These people would perform clerical and housekeeping jobs.

The pre-professionals are aides who have had college training and are apprenticing themselves to a teacher. This differs from student teaching since the college or university is not involved in the training. Pre-professionals have more professional roles than paraprofessionals.

The paraprofessional would be expected to have some formal training and be able to perform some of the tasks that have up to this point been done by a certified teacher.

Furthermore, Anderson contends in some areas the

paraprofessional would be more competent than the teacher and would *only* be useful if this were the case. Paraprofessionals would also be provided with opportunity to get what formal training they needed and to substitute actual experience for a traditional teacher training program.

This view implicitly states the paraprofessional would be competent to replace the teacher in some instances. Bennett and Falk (1970) point out that this position raises many important issues about the supervisory responsibility of the teachers. It is not difficult to understand why there has been confrontations by teachers in several states where this has been implemented. Teachers have been adamant in arguing that non-certified personnel can never assume actual teaching but must always work under the supervision of a certified teacher.

Considering this concern, as well as the greater complexities of the expectations of the teacher's role, Nikolai (1970) proposes a need to better utilize the staff in schools. He views the introduction of paraprofessionals as a better way to utilize staff by dividing them into five categories of responsibility. Each category would require different competency, educational background, and training. Some tasks would require more formal education and a college degree, others perhaps only a week-long inservice workshop. He also pointed out that it would be important to develop stages for career development and a differentiated pay scale so that those who were upwardly mobile would be able to move from step to step.

The categories Nikolai suggested were: 1) technical aides whose responsibilities would be setting up and caring for audio-visual equipment, making transparencies, decorating bulletin boards, and assisting students in learning how to use the equipment; 2) clerical aides who would assist in classroom housekeeping chores, typing and duplicating tests, correcting homework and tests; 3) non-certified instruction aides who would work with students with independent study problems, set up materials for science experiments and work with students under the supervision of the professional teacher; 4) supervisory aides who would supervise recess, behavior and assist on field trips; and 5) community instructional aides whose responsibility would include consulting and making presentations of business, industry and would assist professionals with curriculum revisions.

This model called for the use of a supporting personnel coordinator whose task it would be to see that support personnel were assigned to teachers as the needs for them arose. What makes this approach more palatable for teachers is that a clear differentiation between what paraprofessionals and what teachers do is proposed. The notion of differentiated staffing patterns using paraprofessionals was also proposed by Sharpes (1970), Lawson (1964), Pearl (1968) and Perkins (1966). What was presented to teachers as an opportunity to have more time to teach and, therefore, improve the quality of education had a second aim—that of restructuring the American schools by providing a career ladder. U.S. Commissioner of Education, Harold Howe, stated that the need for the career ladder was urgent in order to institutionalize the aide programs. Therefore, it needed to be built into the program from the beginning (Weisz, 1970). In a sense, then, the teacher's position was threatened to the extent that aides would progress up the ladder and reduce the employment opportunities of the traditionally trained teacher.

As a result of EPDA, 14,000 low income and minority people (88% female) in COP's 132 projects worked as instructional aides in nearly 3,000 public schools. Of these paraprofessionals close to 4,500 completed their degree and found employment as fully certified teachers, usually in the same neighborhood or reservation where they served as aides. This was true despite the nationally publicized oversupply of teachers (Kaplan, 1976). For those who achieved this status it was not only a means of upward mobility for themselves, but also provided an explicit message to the children they worked with that it was possible to climb the ladder.

The COP program provided the potential for getting more personnel into the school and, consequently, provided the opportunity for some students to get more personal attention as well as giving instructors more time to enrich and improve their teaching. Whether this happened, in fact, depended very much on the individual teacher and the structure of the programs.

One of the more successful paraprofessional programs greatly aided by the Career Opportunity Program is in Minneapolis. Not only were paraprofessionals encouraged to participate, but the program was carefully designed, coordinated, and adopted by the Board of Education. It made provisions for training that ranged from instruction for specific jobs and basic education to academic courses as well as specifying a career lattice. This included three categories (School Aide I, School Aide II, and School Assistant) and six salary steps. This structure was further delineated by criteria, for selection, transfer opportunities, definition of tasks, salary schedules and fringes. The paraprofessionals were under a certification program administered by the Civil Service Commission. By requiring paraprofessional certification for each step, the roles were defined and this, in turn, made them less of a threat to the teachers. In addition, the Minneapolis program recognized the concern that was prevalent among teachers that administrators would replace teachers with paraprofessionals in order to save money or in times of personnel crisis. In response to this fear the school district adopted these rules in October, 1967:

1. In the absence of the teacher for any reason, the non-professional may not assume or be assigned the responsibilities reserved for teachers.

2. Non-professionals may not be given independent responsibility for classroom management and organization.

3. The non-professional may not function in a normal classroom helping role if a certified teacher is not available for direction and guidance (Sweet, 1977, p. 116).

There was considerable training of both teachers and paraprofessionals. Teachers were trained to serve as supervisors and evaluators; their professional role has not been compromised.

Although there has been little carefully controlled evaluation done on this program, city-wide testing on reading achievement has increased and paraprofessionals are often in these programs. There was no way of accurately assessing, however, whether this improvement is the result of paraprofessional personnel or if it is the ways in which they have contributed to the improvement. Studies point out that a majority of teachers surveyed by the Minnesota Department of Education perceived that there was a beneficial effect on students' attitude toward school and that the increased individual attention had a positive effect on students' self concept (Sweet, 1977). This, of course, would have more validity if it were carefully evaluated by a well-designed study.

Another consequence of the EPDA was to force teacher training institutions to revise some of their traditional course configurations and go out into the community, providing site-base courses, on-site observations, and active participation in advisory councils in order to make their offerings more relevant (Davies, 1977). As a result, teacher educators were stripped of some of their autonomous power of decreeing the requirements for teacher certification. Rather than making the requirements less stringent, however, the teachers who had consolidated under the auspices of National Education Association, moved to usurp some of the power of the teacher educators and to define for themselves what was necessary to be considered a professional teacher. In a real sense this was a backlash response. Teachers generally welcomed the paraprofessionals who functioned solely to free the teacher of clerical and housekeeping duties. Since it was not always possible to keep teacher aides "in their place," however, teachers as a profession, supported by the National Education Association, have reacted to this movement by introducing legislation that would tighten the requirements for teacher certification. In some states (Michigan, for example), they have gone so far as to push for licensure which will afford them even more protection than certification in that it clearly specifies scope of practice, as well as the make-up of the licensing board (Vlaanderen, 1978).

In summary, the teachers, because of the protection of certification, have used, and will probably continue to use, teacher aides in a narrow way. There is a national movement toward licensure of teachers and since the boards of licensing are likely to be made up of teachers predominately, it appears as if the trend will be to denote clearly what is professional and not allowing anyone to perform in a professional capacity unless they are fully licensed. Insofar as a state makes a commitment to use of paraprofessionals in the schools, it will be urgent that they develop a program similar to the Minneapolis program where role, function, and advancement are carefully specified and teachers are given assurances that paraprofessionals will not pose a threat. At present, there is not much movement in this direction with the exception of a program being designed and implemented in Massachusetts (Glenn, 1977).

*Counselors.*   Guidance has been part of the offerings of the schools since at least 1918. In that year, a pamphlet was issued (Department of Interior, 1918) that asserted that the goal of education was guidance. In defining education and guidance as synonymous, it was implied that those who would provide the guidance were teachers. Crow and Crow (1951) point out that in large elementary schools the position of leading the guidance program was delegated by the principal to a teacher who, in turn, selected teachers to serve as teacher-counselors. In a similar vein, Clendenen (1945) found that in 134 schools in Kansas, in two-thirds of the schools studies, the classroom teacher was assigned the responsibility of providing the guidance function. In other words, there really was no difference in training of the teacher and the counselor and the counselor was simply a teacher who was "annointed" or "appointed" to this role.

In 1958 the National Defense Education Act provided money under Title VA for local school districts to provide better testing programs for secondary school guidance programs. Title VB of the same bill provided for counseling and guidance institutes with stipends for enrollers who wished to become more competent in secondary school counseling (Bernard and Fullmer, 1970). As a result of this, there was a great growth of counselors as evidenced by a growth in membership in the American Personnel and Guidance Association from 18,500 in 1965 (Bernard and Fullmer, 1970) to a present membership of 40,159 as of October 31, 1978.

Despite such a tremendous growth in numbers, however, there seems to be little consensus about how the school counselor defines his/her role and the perceptions of those whom they serve.

The American School Counselor Association approved the Policy for Secondary School Counselors in 1974 when they specified the role of the school counselor:

> Guidance is a function of every member of the educational team, but the responsibility for leadership is one of the primary functions of the school counselor. It assists the student to understand himself by focusing attention on his interests, abilities, and needs in relation to his home, school, and environment. Counseling assists the student in developing decision making competence and in formulating future plans. The school counselor is the person on the staff who has special training for assessing the specific

needs of each student and for planning an appropriate guidance program in the educational, vocational, and personal-social domains. (p. 380)

Typical of students perception are the findings of Van Riper (1971) who reported that:

> The counselor was rather easily identified as a person who helped with educational plans, somewhat identified as a person who helped with school problems, and not clearly identified as a person who helped with personal problems. In addition, the role of the counselor was not easily distinguished from that of the teacher or principal, as evidenced by the large percentage of uncertainty, although there were more students who perceived a role difference than a role similarity. (p. 54)

Teachers generally feel hostile toward counselors and think that they serve no important function and should not be considered a professional in their own right.

> The counselor is a rascal and deserves the admonition that those who teach, teach and those who can't become counselors. A really good counselor teaches at least two periods a day and counsels three, two of which counseling periods he knows in his heart are only prep periods. A full-time counselor is a fraud . . . . (Lewis, 1972 p. 372).

Administrators generally view the counselor as a jack of all trades. Shertzer and Stone (1976) report that many administrators expect the counselors to function as clerks or quasi-administrators and participate in curriculum planning, pupil attendance, schedule making, substitute teaching, and disciplining students. In addition, Hart and Prince (1970) point out the discrepancy between counselors' perception of their roles and that of administrators. They state that many administrators do not believe counselors to be competent to assist students who have personal or emotional problems.

Not only is there great discrepancy between the counselors' view and the populations that he/she deals with directly, but there is at present no right to the title counselor, except in Virginia where a counselor licensing bill has recently been enacted. Often a counselor is a teacher who is endorsed as a counselor on his/her teaching certificate. It is, therefore, not surprising that counselors feel great confusion and insecurity about their role and function in the schools. This is often reflected in their relationship with paraprofessionals.

## Paraprofessionals in School Counseling

The legislation that was responsible for creating teacher-aides was also responsible for providing new approaches and support personnel in the area of counseling. In addition, other legislation such as the Manpower Development and Training Act, the Vocational Education Act, and amendments to the National Defense Education Act made similar provisions for support personnel for the counselor (A.P.G.A., 1967).

As a result of this legislation, the American Personnel and Guidance Association believed it important to issue a policy statement dealing with the role and standards for preparation of paraprofessionals in counseling. The difference between the paraprofessional and the professional counselor was much more clearly specified than the differentiation made by teachers; perhaps another index of the school counselors' role insecurity. The statement read in part:

> Even though agency policy and hiring practices may ultimately determine the actual role of support personnel, the counselor must have a voice in determin-

ing what specific duties can be performed by such personnel. There are certain services, such as the establishment of a formal counseling relationship, for which the counselor must maintain responsibility and which only a counselor can provide. There are certain other services—such as orientation, outreach and recruitment activities, follow-up, development of job readiness, and improvement of personal appearance—which may be more appropriately provided by specially oriented and adequately prepared support personnel. (p. 859)

Interestingly, the introductory remarks of this policy statement clearly state that this does not refer to relationships across professions and intimates that there is a need to do this. This is another indication of the role conflict that Ivey and Robin (1966) discuss. When there is conflict within one's own role it is hard to meaningfully discuss how one relates to other professionals.

The policy statement specified the direct and indirect functions of support personnel. The direct functions include providing information, rapport-building activities, and serving as recorder and observer in small groups. The indirect services deemed appropriate for paraprofessionals were gathering information, making referrals and routine follow-up activities (A.P.G.A.). It was a clearly defined statement of the appropriate and expected role of support personnel.

At the same time, others (Fisher, 1968; Schlossberg, 1967; Samler, 1968) noted the benefits of using support personnel by freeing the counselor from tasks that were important but routine in nature and could be done adequately by a nonprofessional. In the same vein, Goldman (1967) described a "guidance information technician" who would be primarily responsible for collating and translating information. Hoyt (1970) also classified the responsibilities of support personnel in implementing vocational guidance programs. Despite this large literature dealing with benefits of using paraprofessionals, there is little evidence of them being used in the new careers sense as was intended in the COP programs.

Blaker, Schmidt and Jensen (1971), under the auspices of the Professional Services Commission of the California School Counselors Association, studied the use of counselor-aides in California and found that 86% of the schools did not use counselor-aides. Rather, the counselors responded to the idea of support personnel by developing programs and using peer counselors. The literature is full of descriptions of programs for the training and use of peer counselors (e.g. Ettkin and Snyder, 1972; Hamburg and Varenhorst, 1972; Lobitz, 1972; Varenhorst, 1974). It is interesting and significant to note that in the special issue of the *Personnel and Guidance Journal* (1974) dealing with paraprofessionals, the only article dealing with school counselors' use of support personnel was by Varenhorst describing a training program for peer adolescent counselors.

An explanation for this can be found in the lack of clarity in the role and function of the school counselor. As recently as 1978, an article in the *School Counselor* (Osborne, 1978) details ways in which counselors have failed to clarify their role. This continuing confusion contributed greatly to the avoidance of using counselor-aides. School counselors feared that since many of their activities, which were not congruent with what they saw their role to be, could be competently carried out by counselor-aides and they (the counselors) would put themselves in a position where they jeopardized their own jobs. By using peer counselors, however, they could have many menial tasks accomplished without posing any threat to themselves. To the extent that their role and function is full of discrepancies, it is not surprising that paraprofessionals have had little or no impact on school counselors.

## Administrators

The administrators were the first group in the school's organization to professionalize. They clearly specified the standards for preparation that was necessary to perform in the administrative role (Griffith, 1959). In all states they must hold a teachers certificate as well as have completed a master's degree. North Central Association of Colleges and Schools requires the equivalent of a specialist degree (Woellner, 1978). They have also clearly communicated that their function is to coordinate the efforts of school personnel in order to facilitate the achievement of the schools goals (Shertzer and Stone, 1976). More specifically, Campbell, et al. (1971) state that the four primary activities that school administrators typically perform with the goal of advancing teaching and learning are to: 1) influence the goals and policies of the school building or district, 2) facilitate and supervise the development of programs to achieve the goals specified; 3) develop and coordinate an organization to implement these goals; and 4) procure and manage resources to support the organization and its programs.

There appears to be a great deal of role consistency as far as what the public expects school administrators to do and what they say they do. Therefore, one would expect a great deal of job security. How then have administrators used paraprofessionals?

## Paraprofessionals in Administration

As was stated previously, school administration have security in terms of both role consistency and professionalization. They are also on the top of the educational hierarchy. Since this is the case, there is little opportunity for lay people to work as aides in the career ladder sense. They have mainly been used as clerical help. The closest thing to the use of paraprofessionals in administration is the internship that is part of the requirements for a graduate degree and is, therefore, pre-professional. In practice the internship is generally university sponsored and involves placing the student in an administrative position in a school district under the joint supervision of the local school administrator and university personnel. Basically, then, there have been no inroads in the use of paraprofessionals in administration.

## CONCLUSIONS

What can be said about the use of paraprofessionals in education? The COP program held out the hope for a "bold new approach" that would use low income persons to provide direct services to the schools and at the same time to have the opportunity to advance themselves. Overwhelming evidence has demonstrated that these goals have not been met. As Delworth (1974) states:

> Beyond the personal disillusionment of the paraprofessional, little has come of the premise that paraprofessionals would create a real change in the delivery of human services, especially for minorities, the poor, and women. Many agencies remain as racist, sexist, and elitist as though paraprofessionals had never been involved in their operation. How could so many have had such a limited impact on the agencies in which they worked? What happened? (p. 336)

Part of the answer can be found in the basis of the COP program. It was based on a concept that implied new people trained in different ways would become "new professionals" (Gartner and Riessman, 1974). It is not surprising that the assumption that "we would maintain intact the traditional conceptualizations . . . simply by fitting the nonprofessional into the already existing structure of delivery systems" (Minuchin, 1969) could not work. For one thing, the lack of clarity of just how the paraprofessional would function was never adequately resolved. Perhaps having a more important impact is the threat that this program held for the professionals, who saw their own position threatened, the use of paraprofessionals who could usurp their positions. In addition, they viewed the possibility of losing control of their "guild" as not acceptable. In response to this danger, they responded with great resistance by working to establish more stringent and exclusive licensing.

Although there were a sizable number of teachers who have graduated from the COP program, the majority of the teacher-aides have been hampered in rising by the move to tighten certification and licensing in many states. Since teachers can control their role and function by legislation, they are generally happy to have the services of a teacher-aide as long as the aides stay in their place and have no "delusions" they are professionals.

This position, in turn, had an important rebound effect on the paraprofessionals who had been promised an opportunity to move up the career ladder but found it both frustrating and discouraging when this didn't happen. In a real sense, the implication of the failure of this to occur only strengthened their sense of marginality.

In addition, the conflict that ensued from the values of the lower class workers and the middle class schools, were never adequately confronted and worked through. This only heightened the misunderstanding between professionals and paraprofessionals.

A third dimension that remained adequately resolved was helping teachers develop expertise in the role of the supervisor. The skills necessary to perform as a competent teacher are different from those of a supervisor. This lack of training in supervision made the teachers feel both inadequate and angry that they had to assume yet another burden.

The experiences of using educational paraprofessionals has demonstrated that the paraprofessional could provide many useful services as well as serving as a role model to lower class children, but the necessary steps to change the basic structure of the school to accommodate them and address the important underlying dilemmas has not been carried out. Further, it would be necessary to have a commitment from the professional personnel that this was desirable and to devise a way of controling the functions the paraprofessionals could perform. In this era of tight money, falling enrollments, and increased unionization and guild building of professional groups, this does not seem likely to happen.

## REFERENCES

Allen, D. A differentiated staff: Putting teaching talent to work. In Olivero and Buffie *Educational Manpower.* Bloomington, Ind.: Indiana University Press, 1970.

American Personnel and Guidance Association. Support personnel for the counselor: Their technical and non technical roles and preparation. *Personnel and Guidance Journal,* 1967, *45,* 857-861.

Anderson, R. *Teaching in a World of Change.* New York: Harcourt, Brace and World, Inc., 1966.

Announcement and Prospectus of the Training of Teachers and Related Personnel, *New Careers Newsletter* March 13, 1968.

Bennett, W. & Falk, R. *New Careers and Urban Schools.* New York: Holt, Rinehart and Winston, 1970.

Bernard, H., & Fullmer, D. *Principles of guidance: A basic text.* Pennsylvania International Textbook Co., 1970.

Blaker, K., Schmidt, M. & Jensen, W. Counselor-aides in guidance programs. *The School Counselor,* 1971, *18* (5), 382-386.

Bowman, G. & Klopf, G. *New career and roles in the american school.* New York: Bank Street College of Education, 1967.

Campbell, R., Bridges, E., Corbally, J., Nystrand, R., & Ramseyer, J. *Introduction to educational administration*, (4th ed.). Boston: Allyn and Bacon, 1971.

*Career opportunities program.* U. S. Department of Health, Education and Welfare, Office of Education, 1970.

Carter, W. T. The career opportunities project; A summing up. In Gartner, A., Riessman, F., and Jackson, V., *Paraprofessionals Today*, Vol. 1, New York: Human Sciences Press, 1977.

Carter, Barbara and Dapper, Gloria. *School Volunteers— What They do How They Do It.* New York: Citation Press, 1972.

Clendenen, D. A Study of guidance activities of 134 secondary schools of Kansas. Masters Thesis, Syracuse University, 1945.

Crow, L., & Crow, A. *An Introduction to Guidance.* New York: American Book Co., 1951.

Davies, D. Educations Professions Development Act: An inside perspective. In Gartner, A., Riessman, F., & Jackson, V. *Paraprofessionals Today*, Vol. 7. New York: Human Sciences Press, 1977.

DeLaVergne, M. & Blitz, H. Back to class as a teacher aide. *Occupations Outlook Journal*, 1975, *19*(4), 23-25.

Delworth, U. Paraprofessionals as guerillas; Recommendation for system change. *Personnel and Guidance Journal*, 1974, *53*, 335-338.

Denemark, G. *Higher Education National Field Task Force on the Improvement and Reform of American Education.* Washington: American Association of Colleges for Teacher Education, 1974.

Department of Interior. Cardinal principles of secondary education. *Bureau of Education Bulletin No. 35.* Washington, D. C.: Government Printing Office, 1918.

Ettkin, L., and Snyder, L. A model for peer group counseling based on role playing. *The School Counselor,* 1972, *19* (4), 215-218.

Fisher, J. Subprofessionals in pupil personnel services. *National Association of Secondary School Principals Bulletin, 1968, 52,* 49-57.

Ford Foundation. *Decade of experiment: 1951-61.* New York: The Fund for the Advancement of Education, 1961.

Gartner, A. & Riessman, F. The paraprofessional movement in perspective. *The Personnel Guidance Journal,* 1974, *53* (4), 253-256.

Glenn, Charles. *Recommendations on paraprofessional staff.* Boston: Bureau of Educational Opportunity, 1977.

Goldman, L. Help for the counselor. *Bulletin of the National Association of Secondary School Principals,* 1967, *51,* 48-53.

Griffith, D. *Administrative Theory.* New York: Appleton, 1959.

Hamburg, B. & Varenhorst, B. Peer counseling in the secondary schools: A community mental health project for youth. *American Journal of Orthopsychiatry,* 1972, *42*(4), 566-581.

Hart, D. & Prince, D. Role conflict for school counselors: Training vs. job demand. *Personnel and Guidance Journal,* 1970, 48, (5), 374-380.

Hoyt, K. B. Vocational guidance for all: New kinds of personnel needed. *American Vocational Journal,* 1970, *45,* 62-65.

Ivey, A., and Robin, S. Role theory, role conflict and counseling: A conceptual framework. *Journal of Counseling Psychology,* 1966, *13,* (1), 29-37.

Kaplan, G. The career opportunities program: EPDA as mid-range demonstration. *Journal of Teacher Education,* 1976, *27* (2), 148-150.

Kehas, C. Education and personal development. In B. Shertzer, S. Stone, (eds.) *Introduction to guidance: Selected reading.* Boston: Houghton Mifflin, 1970.

Lawson, E. Role of the auxiliary: Teaching in the truest

sense. *Times Education Supplement,* No. 1, 2587, 1964.

Lewis, F. Some of my best friends are counselors. *Phi Delta Kappan,* 1972 *53,* (6), 372-373.

Lobitz, W. Maximizing the H.S. counseling effectiveness: The use of senior tutors. *The School Counselor,* 1972, *19,* 9.

Lucien, B. *Measure of a good teacher.* Sanford, Calif.: California Teachers Association, 1952.

Minuchin, S. The paraprofessional and the use of confrontation in the mental health field. *American Journal of Orthopsychiatry,* 1969, *39* (5), 726.

Moser, R. & Sprinthall, N. Psychological education: A means to promote personal development during adolescence. *The Counseling Psychologist,* 2:4, 1971, *4,* 8-9.

National Education Association. *Teacher aides in large school systems.* Washington, D. C.: Association of Educational Research Service, 1967.

Nikolai, I. Differential personnel: A rational. In J. Olivero, & F. Buffie. *Educational Manpower.* Bloomington, Ind.: Indiana University Press, 1970.

Osborne, W. I'd like to try that, but . . . . *The School Counselor,* 1978 *5,* 342-345.

Pearl, A. New careers and the manpower crisis in education. In F. Riessman, & H. Popper, *Up From Poverty.* New York: Harper and Row, 1968.

Pearl, A. & Riessman, F. *New careers for the poor.* New York: Free Press, 1965.

Perkins, B. How to use teacher aides effectively. *Getting better results from teacher aides, substitutes and volunteers.* Englewood Cliffs, N.J.: Prentice Hall, 1966.

Ryan, K. A plan for a new type of professional training. In Olivero, J. and Buffie, F. *Educational Manpower.* Bloomington: Indiana University Press, 1970.

Samler, J. Vocational counseling: A pattern and a projection. *Vocational Guidance Quarterly,* 1968, *17,* 2-11.

Schlossberg, N. Subprofessionals: To be or not to be.

*Counselor Education and Supervision,* 1967, *6,* 108-113.

Sharpes, D. A model of differentiated teaching personnel. In J. Olivero & E. Buffie. *Educational Manpower.* Bloomington, Ind.: Indiana University Press, 1970.

Shertzer, B. & Stone, S. *Fundamentals of guidance.* Boston: Houghton Mifflin Co., 1976.

Sub-Professional Career Act, *Title II, Section 205e,* 1966 and *Title I-B, Section 123 of Equal Employment Opportunity Act* of 1967. Washington, D.C.: U.S. Government Printing Office.

Sweet, A. A decade of paraprofessional programs in the Minneapolis public schools. In A. Gartner, F. Riessman, & V. Jackson, *Paraprofessionals Today,* Vol. 1.

Tanner, L. & Tanner, D. The teacher aide: A national study of confusion. *Educational Leadership,* 1969, *26, 8,* 765-772.

The American School Counselor Association. The role of the secondary school counselor. *The School Counselor,* (May, 1974), *21,* 380.

VanRiper, B. Student perception: The counselor is what he does. *The School Counselor,* (September, 1971), *19,* 54.

Varenhorst, B. Training adolescents as peer counselors. *Personnel and Guidance Journal,* 1974, *53* (4), 271-275.

Vlaanderen, R. State review: Program report on teacher certification programs around the country. *Education Commission of the States,* Nov. 1978, *43,* 4-5.

Weisz, V. Auxiliary personnel in education. In J. Olivero, & E. Buffie, *Educational Manpower.* Bloomington, Ind.: Indiana University Press, 1970.

Woellner, E. *Requirements for certification.* Chicago: University of Chicago Press, 1978.

# Paraprofessionals in Criminal Justice

Joseph E. Scott,
*Department of Sociology,*
*The Ohio State University*

With public attention focused on high crime and recidivism rates, the field of corrections in recent years has been more willing to investigate various alternative programs for crime prevention and control. One area receiving considerable attention has been the use of indigenous paraprofessionals.

Although utilization of paraprofessionals in the criminal justice professions has often been described as being related to personnel shortages (Korn, 1968, p. 73; Gartner, 1971, pp. 9-11) several alternative arguments have been advanced. Scott (1975, pp. 59-64) argued that paraprofessionals' primary contribution was in bridging the gap between middle class professionals and their clients. Cressey (1965, pp. 57-59) and Empey (1971) both maintained that the use of paraprofessionals in criminal justice would provide better services to clients and provide new job opportunities for an otherwise "exploited class" in our society. Bullington, Munns and Geis (1969, pp. 458-461) suggested the use of paraprofessionals in criminal justice gave such individuals an opportunity to better themselves while at the same time assuring the community that criminal justice practitioners were willing to do what they were requesting of the rest of society, namely, give ex-offenders an opportunity for self betterment through job opportunities. Whatever the salient reasons may be, the use of paraprofessionals and more specifically the use of ex-offenders in criminal justice has become much more a reality during the last decade.

Paraprofessionals, under various titles and roles, were participating in New Deal programs as early as 1935, but it was not until the 1960s that they gained widespread popularity. The modern paraprofessionals made their first major debut in the school system. The health agencies and other social service agencies quickly followed in the use of paraprofessionals. These first programs recruited largely middle-class persons to supplement the work of the trained professionals (Gartner, 1971).

With the black, civil rights, antiwar, and student movements of the 1960s, a new awareness of human rights exploded on the American scene. A greater demand for more and a better quality of life combined with a new element of community identification and community control met head on with the existing manpower resources. Many believed there were simply too few workers with the traditional social-biographical background and abilities to meet the new demand. Thus, a shift to a new type of manpower evolved—a man with definite community ties but less formal training. Reiff and Riessman (1970, p. 7) saw this new worker as a "peer of the client who shares a common background, language, ethnic origin, style and common interest." The indigenous paraprofessional, therefore, was born almost overnight.

The most obvious use of the indigenous paraprofessional is to increase service efficiency and effectiveness. This is done most frequently in two ways: by relieving the professional of time-consuming tasks that require little special training, and by providing new services not offered by the professional. It is within this second realm that the indigenous paraprofessional makes his special contribution to the service agency. The indigenous paraprofessional without formal training is capable of doing this because of his desire to be of service and his close community ties. These traits are especially helpful in dealing with minority and ethnic groups of which the professional may not be a member. Likewise, the indigenous paraprofessional is in an ideal position to influence the existing attitudes of the professionals concerning the members of the community, thus enabling the professional to deal more effectively with those he serves.

Where most paraprofessionals were nonindigenous personnel, they were viewed as handmaidens of the professionals with whom they worked. There is a marked difference in the way in which indigenous personnel are viewed today. They are hired because of the unique contributions they can make to the local community and to the agency in which they work. Research by Carkhuff and Truax (1965, pp. 426-432) and Scott (1975, p. 98) indicates that nonprofessionals can be as effective as trained professionals in dealing with most problems and people. Consequently, recent programs using indigenous workers have given these paraprofessionals major responsibilities in servicing client needs in the human services area.

Widespread use of indigenous workers within agencies and organizations began in the early 1960s. The first major programs were funded under the President's Committee on Juvenile Delinquency and Youth Crime. MFY (Mobilization for Youth), located in New York City's Lower East Side, used indigenous persons in school and community work. This program lead Riessman (1963) to publish his first call for what he called "the new non-professional."

In 1964, with the Economic Opportunity Act and the launching of the Office of Economic Opportunity (OEO), an increasing demand for the indigenous paraprofessional arose. The rash of new programs called for more and better services for the poor, and at the same time provided an opportunity for employment of these same people. After the first year, OEO employed 25,000 paraprofessionals in community-action programs and almost twice that number in the Head Start Program (Schmais, 1967, p. 7).

By the late 1960s, with new and modified legislation, indigenous paraprofessionals had become a fact of life in the labor force. Not only did their numbers increase, but their effectiveness became less disputable. Pearl and Riessman (1965) pinpointed even earlier the reasons for the paraprofessionals' potential success. They maintain that the paraprofessional, as a peer of those he serves, becomes a "significant other" in the lives of his clients. Likewise, as a member being served by the community, the paraprofessionals had "inside" knowledge about the workings of the community.

## Ex-Offender Volunteer and Self-Help Programs

It is little wonder with the attention paraprofessionals received by the press and academicians and the apparent success and development of paraprofessional programs that the criminal justice agencies began to explore the possibility of such programs. The initial programs apparently used offenders and ex-offenders as volunteers rather than paid paraprofessionals.

In 1964, two programs were begun within correctional facilities. The Draper Project, conducted at the Draper

Correctional Center in Elmore, Ala., was a unique approach to vocational and educational training. The project initiated a training program to be run solely by inmates, with many prisoners producing self-instructing educational materials (McKee, 1964, pp. 174-176).

The Massachusetts Correctional Institution at Walpole developed a similar program, where prisoners were encouraged to prepare instructional materials for their own use as well as for use by handicapped children and youth. The program, began under the direction of Dr. Harold Ruvin of the Department of Special Education of the Boston University School of Education, and is currently cailed "The New England Materials for Instruction Center" (Inmates of Massachusetts Correctional Institution, 1969).

In 1964, Baker, associate warden of the federal prison at Terre Haute, Indiana, reported on the use of inmate self-government programs throughout the United States in the *Journal of Criminal Law, Criminology, and Police Science* (Baker, 1964, pp. 39-47). Results of his study showed unsuccessful attempts at self-government at 13 institutions. Baker noted that the major problem of such programs was their use of inmates as disciplinarians. Baker proposed the use of inmate advisory councils as a workable alternative, to permit inmates the opportunity to take a more active and constructive role in the improvement of the prison environment while avoiding the difficult role of a disciplinarian.

The most characteristic element of these early programs was the active involvement of the inmate in self-help or self-improvement activities. Later programs moved a step further by using the offender and ex-offender in helping not only himself but others, especially members of his peer group.

Numerous other inmate counseling projects began in the 1960s in several institutions such as the Colorado State Penitentiary (BARS Project), San Quentin (Squires' Program), and the Massachusetts Correctional Institution at Walpole (Project Youth). The focus in all of these programs was helping the youthful segment of the community, especially those singled out as potential offenders. Inmates meet with the juveniles and interested adults to share personal experiences and counsel potential delinquents about the disadvantages of antisocial behavior (Morris, 1970).

In a somewhat different vein, the North Carolina Prison Department began a joint venture with the Institute of Government at the University of North Carolina, called the Chapel Hill Youth Development and Research Unit (CHYDARU). It was a camp for young felons transferred from the state penitentiary, and was staffed entirely by parolees (Keve, 1967, p. 212).

About this same time, Synanon Foundation began assisting a small prison camp on Peavine Mountain, north of Reno, Nevada. The Synanon groups visited the prisoners three times a week to conduct discussion sessions or participate in recreational activities. Members of the Synanon group were, themselves, former inmates (Keve, 1967, p. 216).

In 1969, the Norfolk Fellowship (a program bringing community members into the Massachusetts Correctional Institution at Norfolk to attend fellowship meetings with inmates) began Project Re-entry. The program allowed ex-offenders who had "made it" on the outside to return to the prison and offer their experience and insights to men ready for release. After 4½ years of experience, the program proved to be quite successful, and the ex-offender was viewed by both prison officials and prisoners as a valuable resource (Morris, 1970, pp. 6-7).

One of the best known self-help programs staffed by ex-offenders is the Seventh Step Program, begun at the Kansas state prison as a prerelease program for inmates who were within four months of their release date. In 1965, the first facilities for helping released inmates began with the purpose of aiding convicted offenders to reestablish themselves in the community. Today, the program extends from New York to California, aiding the ex-convict in finance, employment, housing, and friendship (Sands, 1967).

A number of groups have been formed by ex-offenders to provide service and support to offenders. Unlike the Seventh Step Foundation, which is nationwide, most of these other groups are local. The Future Association of Alberta, Canada is one such group which offers a friendly atmosphere where previously incarcerated persons can meet people and make new friends who share common fears and problems. The Self Development Group located in the Deer Island House of Correction in Boston and the Massachusetts Correctional Institution at Concord provide discussion groups and support to ex-offenders and avoid the use of professionals (e.g. social workers, psychiatrists and counselors). Efforts From Ex-Convicts (EFEC) located in Washington, D.C. was organized primarily as a job referral service by ex-cons for ex-cons. EFEC along with a number of other ex-convict organizations is reportedly to be considering publishing a national directory of all such groups as a guide to ex-offenders desiring to work. They plan to stay involved in helping offenders with problems (Goldfarb and Singer, 1973, pp. 598-604; EFEC, Note 1).

The House of Judah in Atlanta and Youth Development, Inc. are two additional community programs run by ex-convicts that attempt to provide service to youth in the area. The former focuses on juvenile runaways and drug users, the latter, addresses itself to teenagers exhibiting antisocial behavior (Sagarin, 1969).

In the area of law enforcement, indigenous workers who have been involved in police-community-relations programs have also met with success. Of particular note is a program initiated by the Los Angeles Police in 1965 shortly after the Watts riots. The indigenous workers employed by the department were all school dropouts, and 75% were ex-offenders. They participated in community activities and aided police in crime and narcotic prevention (Los Angeles Police Department, Note 2).

Unlike the true paraprofessional programs, however, the initial programs in criminal justice cited above mostly offered voluntary or low-paying jobs for the offenders and ex-offenders. The major attribute lacking in such programs was continuing career possibilities in the helping field. Not until the development of the New Careers program in 1967 was the full potential of paraprofessionals in corrections realized. Rather than just providing supplementary helpers or volunteers, the New Careers program offered permanent jobs and a career-ladder concept of paraprofessionals. This new direction occurred by an important amendment to the Economic Opportunity Act in 1966. The New Careers program probably did more than any other effort to insure the use of offenders as paraprofessionals in the field of corrections. It also changed the direction of using offenders as "correctional resources" by providing them with meaningful new careers. Empey (1968) pointed out some of the implications for corrections:

> Our overriding concern is with new careers for offenders, not just with using offenders as a correctional resource. They are already being used as a resource. Our task now is to integrate that use into a larger scheme in which, by being of service to corrections, they might realize lasting career benefits. (p. 6)

The field of corrections was ripe for the New Careers program. As Clements indicated in his handbook for parole officer aides, public attention has tended to focus on rising crime rates and punishment of the offender rather than on rehabilitation. Concomitantly, a critical problem exists in the administration of criminal justice in trying to adequately supervise and help offenders modify their behavior and conform to conventional standards. The social distance between the correction workers and the offenders has often been suggested as one of the major problems, resulting in recidivism and even higher crime rates (Clements, 1972).

## STATES' USE OF EX-OFFENDER PARAPROFESSIONALS IN CORRECTIONS

In 1968, the Joint Commission on Correctional Manpower and Training (1968, pp. 88-90) published a report on the employment of offenders and ex-offenders in correctional work in the United States. The report was based on responses from state adult and juvenile central offices, institutions, and probation and parole agencies. Of 71 responding offices, 66 indicated they could hire offenders and ex-offenders. Only 22, however, reported any such employees. The Joint Commission's report on 461 adult and juvenile institutions throughout the United States reported only 45 with one or more ex-offenders employed in any type of program. Finally, of the 49 state parole agencies, seven state probation agencies and 42 state parole and probation agencies combined responding to the survey, only 15 reported, as of March 1, 1967, having any ex-offenders as employees. One conclusion from this survey is that there are few ex-offenders working as employees of state correctional agencies. Moreover, the reason was not generally because of legal or policy restrictions, but apparently the lack of commitment on the part of state correctional employees to the desirability of such programs.

California, an exception to these findings, began the Parole Service Assistant Program in 1965, to provide job opportunities to hardcore unemployed and to improve the quality of parole services. More than 300 paraprofessionals have worked in the department. By July, 1968, parole aides had become liaisons between the paroles and the parole officer (New Careers Development Project, 1968).

In 1971, Project MOST (Maximizing Oregon's Services and Training for Adult Probation and Parole) used three ex-offenders as paid aides performing assignments at a paraprofessional level. They helped remove professional staff from routine, time-consuming activities (Chandler and Lee, 1972).

Between October, 1968 and September, 1972, a two-phase program using paraprofessional probation officer assistant (POAs) was initiated and supervised by the University of Chicago's Center for Studies in Criminal Justice and the U.S. Probation Office for the Northern District of Illinois (Chicago). This project utilized 52 part-time indigenous workers of whom 22 were ex-offenders. The POAs, under the supervision of professionally trained probation officers, provided direct services for probationers and parolees (Pilcher, Witkowski, Rest, and Busiel, 1972). Members of the project advisory committee were so impressed with the results of the program that they recommended to the Judicial Conference Committee on Probation the creation of permanent full-time paraprofessional positions in the U.S. probation offices. The Judicial Conference endorsed the idea and budgeted 50 such positions for fiscal 1973; congress appropriated money for 20. Gordon (1976, p. 105) found that these paraprofessionals "could provide valuable services to most, if not all, of the clients in the probation system."

Although, as one can see, the concept of using ex-offenders as paraprofessionals in the criminal justice system received considerable attention throughout the 1960s and early 1970s, it apparently was more of an ideal than a reality. As indicated by the Joint Commission on Correctional Manpower and Training's report, very few states had programs for ex-offenders. One of the most ambitious such programs began in Ohio in 1972 (Scott, 1975).

## OHIO'S PAROLE OFFICER AIDE PROGRAM

The Ohio program, the Parole Officer Aide Program began in September, 1972 under the auspices of the state's Adult Parole Authority. Its purpose was to use ex-offenders as quasi-parole officers with their own case loads. During the first year of operation, 13 ex-offenders were hired as aides; an additional 10 were employed in the second year bringing the total number of ex-offender parole officer aides (POAs) in Ohio to 23 by 1973.

From its inception, the Ohio Parole Officer Aide Program was carefully monitored and evaluated to determine the effectiveness of ex-offenders as quasi-parole officers. A control group of parole officers was selected to compare their work and effectiveness to the POAs'. Supervisors, fellow parole officers, parolees, inmates and others were contacted over a three year period to determine the effectiveness of the POA program. The results (although cited by LEAA as an exemplary project) were less than overwhelming. Although resistance to the program quickly diminished and the POAs' work was comparable on almost every indicator examined to that of the parole officers, the recidivism rate of parolees supervised by aides was not significantly different than those supervised by "regular" parole officers.

The most apparent result of the project was the absorption of middle class values by the POAs. The aides were apparently coopted into respectable society, concomitant with a change in their self-image. A number of POAs expressed considerable painful conflict between their old and new roles and generally chose to minimize this by increased efforts on behalf of their parolees. The author's observations suggested that this conflict was intense and that in order to put distance between themselves and their parolees, it was necessary for them to become even more conforming to agency expectations than typical parole officers. The author's conclusion was that an ex-offender's effectiveness stemming from being an Ex-offender Parole Officer Aide diminished with his time in the program. His co-optation was quick and effective in making him a middle class law abiding individual.[1]

## NATIONAL SURVEY OF STATES' USE OF EX-OFFENDERS IN PAROLE AND PROBATION WORK

In 1973, the National Advisory Commission on Criminal Justice Standards and Goals (1973, pp. 478-479) urged correctional agencies to actively hire ex-offenders to work in an assistants' capacity with convicted offenders. One possible reason for their strong endorsement of this policy was that many practitioners claimed that the movement in the area of corrections was more rhetorical than operable. Information about the actual number and types of programs in various state correctional agencies had not been gathered since the Joint Commission Survey in 1967. The lack of such data may have been an inhibiting factor for some states to move forward and implement such programs. One state director of corrections commented: "We hear all the time about the great potential of ex-offender programs for corrections, but we never see any data on who's using them and what the results are."

As part of the Ohio's Parole Officer Aide evaluation, an attempt was made to compile a current and complete survey of the types and numbers of indigenous paraprofessional (ex-offender) programs being used in the nation, especially in the areas of probation and parole. The survey of the use of ex-offenders in corrections began in March, 1974. The purpose of the survey was to gather baseline data about the use of ex-offender paraprofessionals, as well as various attitudes toward the use of such

[1]A similar point is made by Riley et al. in their study of paraprofessionals in CMHCs (Editors).

indigenous workers. Mailed responses were received from 48 of the 51 polled administrators. The remaining three state directors were contacted by telephone and interviewed. The multiple answers that were received, (some state directors circulated the questionnaire to other agencies, such as halfway houses, etc.) were simply averaged together to assign an overall response from that state. On questions dealing with parole and probation, the decision was made to report only the responses received from the various state directors of corrections, unless the state director of probation was the principal respondent. Also, since several of the states have decentralized probation programs and no one individual knows the entirety of activities in the field of probation, data on the use of ex-offenders as parole officers or aides were emphasized.

It was unquestionably difficult for many state directors of corrections to respond accurately to whether their state used ex-offenders as parole or probation officers and aides. One of the major reasons for this difficulty was simply that in at least nine states, there are no legal or administrative restrictions prohibiting ex-offenders from state employment. Consequently, several directors maintained, little effort is made to document whether correctional employees have criminal records or not.

A total of 16, or approximately 33%, of the states reported the use of ex-offenders as parole officers or aides. In 10 or almost 25% of the states responding ex-offenders were used as probation officer aides. The number of such employees range from one such employee in five states to 23 in Ohio, and 55 in Pennsylvania. Most states reported having from one to 10 ex-offender employees.

Using former offenders as parole officers is a relatively new phenomenon, as judged by the initial dates given for the initiation of such practices. California began its program in 1967; Washington in 1968; and four states, Alaska, Maryland, Utah, and Wisconsin, report similar programs beginning in 1970. In 1971, four additional states initiated ex-offender parole officer programs; five more states implemented such programs in 1972; and one state reported beginning a program in 1973. Apparently between 1970 and 1972 was the period when most of the programs began. In fact, of the 139 ex-offender parole officer aides employed as of March, 1974, throughout the United States, 117, or more than 48%, are employed in states that initiated their programs during this period. It may be of interest to note that all 13 programs that began between 1970 and 1972 received LEAA funding. Of the ex-offender parole aide programs initiated before this time, only one, of the three, reported federal funding. The tremendous growth and adoption of such programs may, therefore, be an outgrowth of federal interests in supporting such innovations.

The use of probation officer aides has followed a similar line of development and funding as parole officer aides. All but one of the state programs, begun since 1970, received federal funding. Of particular note is that all 10 states with probation officer aide programs also have parole officer aide programs.

## States' Legal and Administrative Restrictions Concerning Employing Ex-Offenders

Several state directors mentioned that one of the motivating factors for initiating their ex-offender parole officer aide program was the need to set an example for other employers to hire ex-offenders. A typical comment was: "The commission cannot ask other employers to consider hiring ex-offenders without first hiring them ourselves." Despite the validity of such logic, administrative or legal restrictions limit the employment of ex-offenders for parole or probation work in 15 states (Hunt, Bowers, and Miller, 1973). A total of 11 state directors of correction report legal restrictions such as:

Parole officers are "peace officers" and must be licensed

to carry firearms, and it is against our state law for a convicted felon to carry a firearm.

The state, county, or municipality may not employ a person convicted of a felony who has not, prior to the time of filing an employment application, received a full pardon.

Our state personnel still refuses to hire if a potential employee has been convicted of a felony or is under felony indictment.

Convicted felons lose their citizenship and cannot be sworn to oath of office until citizenship is restored.

Convicted felons cannot by law be appointed to a position of trust.

A total of nine states reported administrative restrictions limiting the employment of ex-offenders in parole or probation work. In four of these nine states, there were no legal restrictions, only administrative ones.

In addition to legal and administrative restrictions prohibiting ex-offenders' employment in parole and probation work, other factors discourage many ex-offenders from participating in such programs. Low compensation is, no doubt, one determining factor. The average beginning pay for such employees is $483.52 per month, or $5802.21 per year. The highest beginning pay for parole or probation aides is in Alaska, where the lowest starting pay is $687.00 per month, or $8244.00 per year. The pay scale for ex-offenders in parole or probation work is also quite limited. Often aides are unable to advance to higher professional levels and, therefore, their highest earnings are considerably restricted. The highest salaries for ex-offender aides range from $6684 to $16,800 per year with the average maximum salary being $10,352 or $862.67 per month. With such financial barriers and the additional administrative and professional restrictions, aides in some positions may be locked into a low paying job with little hope of advancement within the agency.

Although definite barriers exist in some states, several state and federal agencies actively recruit ex-offenders for their respective parole and probation aide programs, as well as other important positions. For example, several state ombudsmen were formerly ex-offender parole officer aides. At least one assistant prison warden was a former aide, and one administrative assistant to a state director of correctional services is a former offender.

Another positive point of the ex-offender parole and probation programs is the opportunity provided aides for educational advancement. A total of 12 of the 16 states that utilize ex-offenders as parole or probation officer aides provide paid release time from the job for educational advancement. In addition, financial aid is available in at least 11 of the 16 states to defray the educational expenses. Such available support and encouragement may solve the dilemma of low pay by preparing the former offender for better-paying jobs.

## ATTITUDES OF CORRECTIONAL PERSONNEL TOWARD EMPLOYING EX-OFFENDERS AS PEERS

The major question about all ex-offender programs is their level of success. State directors of correction were asked to rank (on a scale of 0 to 100, with 50 being average) the overall job performance of their ex-offender aides compared with regular staff members performing similar tasks. Overall, aides' performance was rated very good for the 16 states, the average being 67.8, with a range from 30 to 100. Aides are apparently judged to be highly effective in those states where they are employed.

Certainly, if the field of corrections is to utilize the ex-offender in a meaningful role, the support of correctional personnel is essential. The Joint Commission on Correctional Manpower's 1967 survey found that more than 50% of the correctional personnel interviewed felt that it would not be a good idea to hire ex-offenders in their agency. The current survey found a definite shift in this respect. A total of 80% of the state directors believed it desirable to hire ex-offenders in their agencies today. Moreover, in those states utilizing ex-offeners as aides, directors were even more complimentary and committed to the idea than in states not using such programs. Although the desirability of such programs between states utilizing and not utilizing ex-offenders are not statistically significantly different, there does appear to be less opposition to such new programs today, even in those states that have not implemented them.

All state directors of corrections were asked to list both the advantages and disadvantages of utilizing ex-offenders as officers or aides. The advantages most often mentioned were the greater rapport ex-offenders were able to develop with parolees and probationers, and the ability of the ex-offenders to empathize with the problems experienced by the parolees and probationers. Directors made such comments as:

They (the offenders) bring with them the unique quality of being on both sides of the correctional process and, thereby, can more readily identify with offenders' fears and problems.

It gives some legitimacy to our requesting employers to consider hiring an ex-offender if we have some on our own staff. It's pretty difficult justifying to a potential employer why he should hire an ex-con if your own agency refuses to hire him.

Finally, an advantage mentioned by a number of directors dealt with the mediating role such employees could perform between parolees and the parole department.

They (ex-offenders) could teach us how parolees think and why they do some of the "crazy" things they do. In addition they could justify many of our policies and rules to parolees in a way that they might accept them. Hell, we can use any help nowadays that we can get, regardless of the source.

The major disadvantages mentioned by state directors of corrections in utilizing ex-offender employees center around negative stereotypes about former offenders. Comments by directors included:

(The professional staff) would be incensed by lowering our selection criteria.

Public support can certainly not be counted on if your office is packed with ex-offenders.

Hiring such undesirables is simply inviting the corruption of your office and clients.

Such reactions tend to support the observation that self-righteousness lies at the core of the public contempt for offenders. Certainly, public opinion can be mobilized, placated, and won over. In the case of the ex-offender, this may be done most efficiently by appeals to the public's self-interest (demonstration of the effectiveness of ex-offenders in working with parolees curbing crime), combined with the reiterated support of societal standards (i.e., everyone should have an equal opportunity to compete). A major deficiency of ex-offenders gaining such public support is their lack of a major spokesman. Without such vocal support, negative public opinion continues and ex-offenders tend to operate from a weak and most vulnerable position.

The 1974 survey of the 50 states and the District of Columbia found considerably more support for using ex-offenders in correctional work than was the case in 1967. Not only did more state favor using such indigenous workers in 1974, but several states had implemented such programs since 1967. Most of the programs implemented since 1967 were supported by federal funding. Whether the states are truly committed to the idea of utilizing ex-offender personnel may be more accurately answered when such federal funding is no longer available.

It does appear that the ex-offender's involvement in corrections may continue to increase, if for no other reason than the phenomenon of "jumping on the band-wagon." Using ex-offenders as parole, probation officers or aides is a relative new idea. Adopting new programs in this area may dissipate some of the recent criticism corrections has received. State directors of corrections where ex-offenders are presently being utilized as probation, parole officers or aides appear much more committed to the desirability of such programs than directors in states where such programs are not in use, although this relationship is not statistically significant (Scott, 1975, p. 87). Whether utilizing ex-offenders in corrections affects state directors' attitudes favorably, or directors already favoring such programs are the ones implementing them, cannot be answered from this data. It is very apparent, however, that utilizing ex-offenders as parole or probation officer aides is considered very desirable today by most state directors of corrections (for a state-by-state breakdown concerning attitudes, use, restrictions and other data on ex-offenders in corrections, see Scott, 1975).

The future role of ex-offenders in correctional work may well be determined by top administrators in the respective state correctional departments. Unless such programs are supported by those in decision-making positions, however, it is unlikely that they will survive for long. There appears to be growing and continuing support for implementing ex-offender programs on a wider basis. This may be simply a reaction to the enormous criticism corrections has received during this decade. It may also be based on the need to provide legitimate job opportunities for ex-offenders and parole departments' realization to take such initiatives if they expect the private sector of society to do so. Their success or failure may also be determined not only by the quality of ex-offenders selected, but also by the support such programs receive from professionals in the field. If professionals accept ex-offenders as complimentary co-workers, as they apparently have in some states, the ex-offender programs are much more likely to be successful. On the other hand, if the professional staff view such new employees as threatening their own positions and compromising the dignity and respect of their agency, such programs will certainly fail.

The use of ex-offenders in corrections is a unique and refreshing approach. Not only does it convey the trust of the state in hiring ex-offenders for responsible positions, but it indicates the willingness of the state to seek new ways to help ex-offenders. Both of these goals are certainly laudable. The growth and acceptance of such programs during the last decade has been remarkable. If the growth and acceptance of such programs continues at the same rate, ex-offender parole officers and aides will be a common and important part of the correctional helping team of the future.

## REFERENCE NOTES

1. Efforts From Ex-Convicts. *Statement of purpose.* Paper, Washington, D.C., 1966. Unpublished paper.
2. Los Angeles Police Department. *An interim evaluation of the community relations aides' performance in the Community Relations Program.* Los Angeles, California, 1969. Unpublished paper.

## REFERENCES

Baker, J. E. Inmate self-government. *Journal of Criminal Law, Criminology and Police Science,* 1964, *55,* 39-47.

Bullington, B., Munns, J. G., & Geis, G. Purchase of conformity: Ex-narcotic addicts among the bourgeosie. *Social Problems,* 1969, *16,* 456-463.

Carkhuff, R. R., & Truax, C. B. Lay mental health counseling: The effects of lay group counseling. *Journal of Consulting Psychology,* 1965, *29,* 426-432.

Chandler, A., & Lee, A. *Final report for Project MOST.* Portland, Ore.: Oregon State Corrections Division, 1972.

Clements, R. D. *Paraprofessionals in probation and parole: A manual for their selection, training, induction and supervision in day to day tasks.* Chicago: University of Chicago, 1972.

Cressey, D. R. Social psychological foundations for using criminals in the rehabilitation of criminals. *Journal of Research in Crime and Delinquency,* 1965, *2,* 44-59.

Empey, L. Offender participation in the correctional process: General theoretical issues. In *Joint Commission on Correctional Manpower and Training, Offenders as a Correctional Manpower Resource.* Washington, D. C.: Superintendent of Documents, U.S. Government Printing Office, 1968.

Empey, L. *Alternatives to incarceration.* Washington, D.C.: Superintendent of Documents, U.S. Government Printing Office, 1971.

Gartner, A. *Paraprofessionals and their performance.* New York: Praeger, 1971.

Goldfarb, R. L. & Singer, L. R. *After conviction.* New York: Simon and Schuster, 1973.

Gordon, M.T. *Involving paraprofessionals in the helping process: the case of federal probation.* Cambridge, Mass.: Ballinger Publishing Co., 1976.

Hunt, J. W., Bowers, J., & Miller, N. *Laws, licenses and the offenders right to work.* Washington, D.C.: National Clearinghouse on Offenders Employment Restrictions and the American Bar Association, 1973.

Inmates of Massachusetts Correctional Institution. Prison days and nights at MCI Walpole. *The Mentor,* July, Walpole, Massachusetts, 1969.

Joint Commission on Correctional Manpower and Training. *Offenders as a correctional manpower resource,* Washington, D.C.: Superintendent of Documents, U.S. Government Printing Office, 1968.

Keve, P. *Imaginative programming in probation and parole.* Minneapolis, Minn.: University of Minnesota Press, 1967.

Korn, R. R. Issues and strategies of implementation in the use of offenders in resocializing other offenders. In *Joint Commission on Correctional Manpower and Training, Offenders as a Correctional Manpower Resource.* Washington, D.C.: Superintendent of Documents, U.S. Government Printing Office, 1968.

McKee, J. Reinforcement theory and the convict culture. *American Correctional Assocation Proceedings,* 1964.

Morris, A. The involvement of offenders in the prevention and correction of criminal behavior. *Massachusetts Correctional Association Bulletin,* 1970, *20,* 6-7.

National Advisory Commission on Criminal Justice Standards and Goals. *Corrections.* Washington, D.C.: Superintendent of Documents, U.S. Government Printing Office, 1973.

New Careers Development Project. *Final Report.* Los Angeles: Institute for the Study of Crime and Delinquency, 1968.

Pearl, A., & Riessman, F. *New Careers for the poor: The Nonprofessional in human service.* New York: The Free Press, 1965.

Pilcher, W. S., Witkowski, G., Rest, E. R., & Busiel, G. J. *Probation officer case aid project, final report, phase II.* Chicago: Center for Studies in Criminal Justice, University of Chicago Law School, 1972.

Reiff, R., & Riessman, F. *The indigenous non-professional, a strategy of change in community action and community mental health programs.* New York: Behavioral Publication, Inc., 1970.

Riessman, F. *The revolution in social work: The new non-professional. Transaction,* 1963, *2,* 12-17.

Sagarin, E. *Odd man in: Societies of deviants in America.* Chicago; Quadrangle Books, Inc., 1969.

Sands, B. *The seventh step*. New York: New American Library, 1967.

Schmais, A. *Implementing nonprofessional programs in human services*. New York: Graduate School of Social Work, New York University, 1967.

Scott, J. E. *Ex-offenders as parole officers*. Lexington, Mass.: D. C. Heath and Co., 1975.

# The Evolution, Current Status and Future of the Alcoholism Counselor's Role

A. M. Schneidmuhl, M.D.,
*Johns Hopkins School of Hygiene and Public Health,
Baltimore, Maryland*

Gloria Doran, M.H.S., and
Irene Jillson, B.A.,
*Regional Training Program for Alcoholism Counselors,
Baltimore, Maryland*

The past 30 years have seen the birth and the rather rapid development of a new professional group, the Alcoholism Counselors. This cadre of front line workers who provide more than 70% of direct patient contact in publicly-funded alcoholism programs, arose from the need of specially-trained and dedicated personnel to deal with a hitherto neglected illness, alcoholism.

In order to gain a better perspective on the current status of alcoholism counseling, we shall briefly trace the development of the profession through time and from various points of view. Moreover, we shall also trace the development of treatment for alcoholism from early beginnings with nonprofessional workers, through the paraprofessional movement that created the alcoholism counselor role and discuss the tasks that have evolved from the role, and what the expectations of these tasks are. Additionally, we shall look at the present practice, how it is done and who is doing it, as well as what future projections can be made regarding salaries, credentialing, and further structuring of the professional role.

## EARLY ATTEMPTS AT TREATMENT

### Lay Therapists

Over the centuries, the effects of alcoholic beverages on human behavior were ill-understood and interpreted in terms of contemporary mores and beliefs; thus, the various epithets designating alcohol and the imbiber (aqua vitae, devils' brew, glutton, poor moral fiber. . . . ) and the corresponding reactions of fear, envy, resentment, and hostility. Lack of understanding regarding the effects of alcohol as well as the reactions evoked in the community were the basis of the punitive and at times, inhumane treatment of the imbiber. It wasn't until the second half of the 18th century that attempts were made to fit excessive drinking and the accompanying complications into a medical model.

As early as 1775, Thomas Trotter at Edinburgh Univ., Scotland, wrote a doctoral thesis titled "Chronic and Continual Drunkenness," describing the condition as a dis-

214 PARAPROFESSIONALS IN THE HUMAN SERVICES

ease, listing the symptoms and outlining a method of treatment. Close to 70 years later (1848) Swedish scientist Magnus Huss coined the words "alcoholism" and "alcohol." In the United States, Benjamin Rush wrote the book *Chronic Drunkenness* in 1802.

Medicine did not accept the challenge, but instead expressed the, then, generally shared idea that the alcoholic is a social or moral deviant and, therefore, outside of medicine's responsibility. E.M. Jellinek, one of the pioneers in the field, helped popularize the medical model of alcoholism. It was only in 1956 that the AMA passed a resolution concerning the "Hospitalization of Patients with Alcoholism" (Journal of AMA, 1956).

The inevitable happened: in the absence of a formal, professional structure to deal with the widespread conditions of distress related to alcoholism, there emerged a group of native or lay healers.

A Baltimore preacher in 1840 converted a group of alcoholics and within 4 to 5 years, the "Washington Movement" had encompassed nearly 500,000 followers. This lay group taught that alcoholism is an illness and that public confession is its cure.

Courtney Baylor, a lay therapist at the Emanuel Church clinic in Boston (1919) and, later, his disciple Richard Peabody (1931) published still reliable experiential material on the treatment and re-education of alcoholics.

In the 1930s, Pierson, a recovering alcoholic, began a system of treatment that had nine steps, very similar to the 12 steps later promulgated by Alcoholics Anonymous (AA).

Common to all these early workers, was an emphasis on an accepting attitude toward the alcoholic patient; accepting him(her) for what he is, and where he is. Without this quality, the alcoholic could not be reached. Moreover, an attitude of hope was essential; a conviction based on common humanity and common potentials. The lay therapist having these qualities seemed to have had success, whatever his/her background or discipline.

## The "Non-professional" Worker

With the founding of AA in 1935 and its rapid success, came the beginning of a successful treatment experience, based on the 12 steps of AA, and practiced by recovering alcoholics working with their peers. The professional community, aware of the success of the AA mutual help model, began to utilize recovering alcoholics in the formal treatment setting. Thus, as early as 1944, AA members, working under the direction and supervision of professionals, provided services at the Yale Clinics in Connecticut. The recovering AA nonprofessional worker brought with him strong motivation to help other alcoholics (12th step work) that was enhanced by the conviction: helping others constitutes part of his own continued treatment program. It was agreed that the recovering AA nonprofessional serves as an example that a break with alcohol is possible. Furthermore, he presented a model of recovery: one who has successfully stopped drinking and was living comfortably. It was also believed that the recovering alcoholic brought to his clients in treatment a wealth of personal experience and a depth of understanding that could not be matched by workers who had not experienced the disease. This point is still a subject of considerable controversy.

The stance of the nonprofessional worker vis-á-vis his client was that of a peer who had experienced the same problem. If the client will follow his example, he too, can master the problem. The emphasis was likely to be on action rather than insight, immediacy rather than considerate study. He was apt to externalize causes and concentrate on problem solving for his client.

Thus, the AA nonprofessional worker was viewed as an adjunct to an established traditional mental health treatment; unfortunately, except for the aforementioned "model role," the adjunctive functions of the nonprofessional were not clearly defined. This created areas of friction between the professionals and the nonprofessionals. Since the authority for treatment decisions rested with the professionals, they viewed themselves as carrying the legal and ethical responsibility for patient welfare while being expected to trust an untrained and unskilled worker to carry out treatment tasks. In many ways, these nonprofessionals were the prototype for the larger paraprofessional movement that emerged in the 1960s.

The emergence of alcohol counselors must be seen in the context of public views on alcohol and alcoholism. In 1944, Marty Mann had founded the National Council on Alcoholism. This is a citizen group dedicated to educating the public that alcoholism is a disease, the alcoholic can be helped and is worth helping, and alcoholism is a public health problem and, therefore, a public health responsibility. By the mid-1940s, several states had laws regarding alcohol education in the schools, and in 1958 the Secretary of HEW publicly named alcoholism as one of the country's four leading health problems. The voters' attitudes toward alcoholism was changing, and there was the start of support for public treatment programming.

The 1960s saw a favorable climate for social legislation, part of the Great Society planning. Alcoholism was linked with crime in the streets and highway traffic safety. In 1966, funds were made available for detoxification units from Department of Justice funds and for counselor training from Model Cities funds. In 1968, the Community Mental Health Center Act was amended to provide services to alcoholics; mental health funding became available for alcoholism. In 1970 congress passed Law 91-616, the so-called Hughes Act, that made provision for Federal funding for alcoholism and established the National Institute on Alcohol Abuse and Alcoholism.

Financial encouragement was given to states to pass the Uniform Act, that defines alcoholism as an illness, thus taking it out of the criminal justice system and categorizing it under public health. Thus, the past 10 years have seen a tremendous expansion in services to alcoholics and consequently demand for trained manpower.

## The Paraprofessional Worker

As previously mentioned, the professionals who were carrying the legal and ethical responsibility for patient welfare were reluctant to trust the untrained and unskilled non-professional to carry out treatment tasks. It was recognized that dedication and personal experience of the AA nonprofessional worker had to be supplemented with some basic practical information about alcohol and alcoholism. Short-term educational programs (such as the Yale Summer School for Alcohol Studies), designed to provide such information and were helped to dispel some misconceptions and myths about alcohol and alcoholism but provided little help in terms of skills and helping techniques. There arose a need for training programs that could provide information about alcohol and alcoholism and, more importantly, promote skills necessary in the ministering to the sick alcoholic and to his environment. It was anticipated that training and team work would convince the professional and the paraprofessional of the therapeutic value of their respective contributions to the program.

During the initial expansion phase of alcoholism treatment facilities, following the infusion of public monies in the late 1960s and early 1970s, there was a need for workers with organizing skills. Agencies needed to be set up, referral sources found, and patients needed to be encouraged to seek treatment. Other community care-givers needed to be educated in the identification and referral of alcohol problems. Thus, in new programs, the role of the counselor was seen as a treatment generalist, a community coordinator and educator, a specialist in establishing referral sources, a case finder. There was little emphasis on therapeutic skills and quality of treatment. As treatment programs became better established, more attention was paid to counseling skills, particularly to group counseling and, more recently, to record keeping.

As a result of training and team-support, the paraprofessional counselor working in these agencies, began to take on further duties: that of group leader, individual counselor, and team worker. In short, the job role was changing from that of an adjunct to the professional treatment team to a full member of the team with interpersonal and organizational awareness.

A survey of graduates of the Johns Hopkins Continuing Education Model for Alcoholism Counselors, conducted in 1974, disclosed that alcoholism counselors were performing the following tasks: case finding; intake and client evaluation; hospital emergency coverage; direct counseling; individual, group, family and crisis intervention; recommendations and arrangements with physicians for medication (antabuse, tranquilizers); education information on alcohol and alcoholism; program administration; client record-keeping; community activities (speaking engagements, workshops, etc.); research. These were reported as the counselors' most frequently performed tasks, and it was apparent that a structured role for alcoholism counselors was emerging from community needs and agency expectations.

Concurrently, others were working on the definition of counselor role. The Roy Littlejohn Associates draft report dated June 18, 1974, listed functional tasks ascribed to alcoholism counselors, and the intent was to develop standards for training and certification. This latter purpose was not accomplished, largely due to resistance on the part of the states to federal standard-setting. The first task, to conduct a survey that described what counselors were actually doing in their jobs, however, was successful. More than 750 agencies, with directors and counselors participating, contributed information to the study.

From the data obtained, a list of 21 task areas and four major competencies was obtained. In addition, a code of ethics was developed to serve as behavioral and attitudinal guidelines for those areas of counselor performance not yet sufficiently defined.

Although the report did not indicate *how much* knowledge was required to do a task, or *how well* the counselor would be expected to do it, it did confirm that: 1) the role of alcoholism counselor was well established; 2) the counselor was expected to perform a broad range of tasks related to the medical, social and psychological needs of his client, and; 3) the major responsibility for treating the "whole person" and coordinating treatment components was in the hands of the alcoholism counselors.

To that point, in attempting to define the role of the counselor, the emphasis had been on what the counselor was called upon to do without any apparent attempt to measure how well he was performing these tasks. In 1974, in conjunction with designing the curriculum content of the alcoholism counselor training program, the staff at Johns Hopkins designed an instrument to measure counselor competencies of student/graduates in the field.

The overall goal of the counselor training program was to train workers competent to fulfill the functions of alcoholism counselors; to provide a pool of trained persons who, by the "ripple" effect, could train others, ultimately raise the quality of patient care, and produce a model program that could be duplicated elsewhere, using program materials and design as well as staff consultation and technical assistance.

Curriculum content was designed around the tasks of the original survey and the Littlejohn Report, providing each trainee (whether experienced or not) with the basic knowledge and skills required to perform the counselor tasks in a variety of treatment settings.

Since job performance standards for counselors were as yet not structured for the alcoholism field, the program developed standards for its students and designed a "Skill Review Instrument" based on behavioral measurement on the job, which could be administered and evaluated by agency supervisors. Performance was measured at the end of didactic training, field placement, and again, six months after graduation.

There were 16 major task areas defined, each rated on a scale of one (excellent) through five (unacceptable) in performance terms. The task areas were; case finding: program administration; diagnosis; intake; treatment plan; individual counseling; group counseling; family counseling; referral services; consultation regarding medication; emergency medical care; crisis intervention; aftercare; record keeping; provision of alcohol information; community activities.

## Current Status

Although the response to the needs of developing alcoholism treatment programs led to the formation of a cadre of trained front-line workers—the paraprofessional alcoholism counselor—political and economic factors have greatly influenced the current trend toward professionalization of this group of workers. In an effort to stimulate states and local agencies to pay for the care of their alcoholic citizens, the federal government has encouraged the inclusion of alcoholism treatment in health insurance policies.

Third party payers, in turn, have requested the development of standards in relation to quality of care, training of personnel, physical plant, and organizational functions. The Joint Commission on Accreditation of Hospitals has agreed to accredit alcoholism treatment agencies, and it is their recordkeeping requirements that both counselors and their agencies have found difficult to fulfill. This in turn, has generated demand for including detailed record keeping in counselor training.

The anticipation of National Health Insurance has

also had an impact on alcoholism counselors roles. Increasingly, alcoholism is viewed as "another" illness, treated by a specialty team, part of an integrated health care system where the alcoholism counselor is an important contributing member.

## CHARACTERISTICS OF THE ALCOHOLISM COUNSELOR

The following composite picture of the alcoholism counselor is based on our experience in the field, as well as on a survey of graduates of our training program.

Typically, the counselor is between 35 and 40 years of age, and has had some college level course work. Men and women are almost equally represented in the field. The worker has usually attended a summer institute or weekend workshops on alcoholism, received some in-service training, and is planning to continue training in the future. He or she has been in the field of alcoholism for less than five years, but plans to remain.

Previous jobs held by these people covered a wide range of vocations, with about one in four coming from other human service settings such as hospital, nursing, social or community work.

Salaries tend to be rather low, with the median being in the $10,000 to $15,000 per annum range. Salary range depends on the location of the treatment setting (urban or rural, private industry or hospital, public clinic, etc.) and functions of the worker; for example those counselor positions which include some administrative duties are better paid than those including only counseling.

Where alcoholism counseling positions have been classified into State or local Health Department salary scales, they tend to compare with those of beginning social workers or nurses, but with less opportunity for advancement. Improvement of alcoholism counselor salary scales is anticipated with certification and third party coverage.

Less than half of the counselors practicing in the field

have had personal experience with alcohol or other drug abuse, and classified themselves as "recovering."

Many others were drawn to the field through family involvement in the disease. Some younger counselors were interested in alcoholism as a specialty area, to enhance a more general practice of counseling, nursing, or probation.

## FUNCTIONS OF THE ALCOHOLISM COUNSELOR

The functions that the alcoholism counselors will be expected to perform and the corresponding skills that he/she will require depend on factors such as work setting, size of the program, size of the staff, philosophy of the agency's program, etc. For example, a counselor in a small rural health department may be the only alcoholism worker and may require all the 16 skills to perform his duties, although another counselor, employed in an emergency room of a metropolitan hospital, may have to specialize in crisis intervention, diagnosis or intake, and may very seldom be called upon for group counseling, educational presentations and the like.

In order to provide for counselor mobility (both upward and lateral) the counselor must have a basic grounding in all the 16 skills.

The following is a brief description of the skills as identified by the staff of the Regional Training Program for Alcoholism Counselors.

1. *Intake*—The intake worker obtains information for the records, gives the patient the opportunity to express why he came for treatment, communicates hope, and encourages the patient to return.
2. *Diagnosis*—Although an official diagnosis of alcoholism must be made by a physician, the counselor can discriminate between psychological and physiological symptomatology, take drinking his-

tories, recognize the stages of alcoholism, and is sensitive to signs regarding "major" or "minor" mental illness. The counselor should be in a position to make diagnostic recommendations regarding alcoholism.

3. *Treatment Plan*—The counselor should be able to formulate, together with client, an individualized treatment plan. This includes long- and short-range goals, and is regularly updated.

4. *Knowledge about Medication*—He/she should be familiar with the commonly-used drugs in treatment of alcoholism, and be able to accurately report their effects on the individual client to the medical staff.

5. *Individual Counseling*—Regarding individual treatment, the counselor must be able to establish a supportive, empathetic relationship with the client, communicate accurate information regarding the illness of alcoholism and its treatment, help the client clarify his/her goals in seeking treatment, and help him/her understand and change his/her use of alcohol in coping with life stresses.

6. *Group Counseling*—This has proved to be most effective in the treatment of alcoholism, as well as being economical. The alcoholism counselor needs to be able to recognize and practice group techniques, maintain group limits, further therapeutic goals, and anticipate and handle group crisis.

7. *Family Counseling*—Alcoholism has been called the "family disease," because the illness impacts on family relationships and is destructive to the psychological well-being of all persons within the family structure. Increasingly, there has been emphasis on treatment of the whole family, and counselors should be able to facilitate communication between family members and assist the family in problem solving.

8. *Referral Services*—Depending on the type of al-

coholism agency, and on the comprehensiveness of the service components, the client may be referred to other agencies. The counselor should have good working relationships with agencies, ideally on a person-to-person level, and be able to follow-up on the referral in some way.

9. *Community and Patient Education*—In most agencies, staff are called on to fulfill two educational functions: to make informational presentations on alcohol and alcoholism, to the patients, and community groups. As in other chronic conditions, the alcoholic patient must learn to manage his/her condition (disease), which involves changes in the patients attitudes, life-style, and behavior. In making these changes, educational/informational sessions can be invaluable.

Community education is necessary for prevention, out-reach, public relations and community organization. In order to be an effective educator, the counselor not only needs a good knowledge of his subject, but must have some planning and presentation skills that can make his educational efforts appropriate and effective in a variety of group settings.

10. *Community Activities*—In small rural communities, the counselor may need to know key civic and community service personnel, in order to raise funds and develop resources. In larger or more urban settings, this responsibility might rest with agency administrators, rather than counselors.

11. *Crisis Intervention*—Counselors in all settings need to be able to operate in crisis situations, to handle intoxicated individuals even when they are physically unruly, and to deal with distressed family.

12. *Aftercare*—Also, in all work situations, counselors must be aware of the need for aftercare of clients, structuring post-treatment contact, and anticipat-

ing possible critical situations when re-contact might be important to the clients current status.

13. *Emergency Medical Care*—As mentioned before, counselors working in an emergency room setting need more medical knowledge than the counselor-generalist. All counselors, however, need to be able to recognize signs of impending delirium tremens, hallucinations, heart failure, seizures, or toxic states. He/she should also have contact with personnel in emergency facilities, and be able to follow up with client post-referral.

14. *Record Keeping*—With the development of standards of care, and the accreditation of agencies, there has been greater and greater emphasis on record keeping. Since the counselor, in nearly all treatment settings, spends more time in direct contact with the patient than any other member of the team it is on him that the primary responsibility for records depends. In accordance with current standards, all counselors should be able to maintain complete and current records, and to develop treatment plans.

15. *Case Finding*—Once again, case finding skills will be more useful in a small agency than in a busy urban setting. Every counselor, however, should be aware that in some job settings it may be necessary to stimulate referrals to the agency and that each worker must play an active part in facilitating referrals and entry of new cases.

16. *Program Administration*—Most treatment agencies function on the team concept, that is, no one individual is solely responsible for patient care. The counselor, therefore, should be aware of the roles and functions of the various workers in the agency, know the organization of the agency and ideally, be able to take on some functions of other workers should the occasion demand it.

The worker needs to know his place in the system and how the system works. He also needs to view his own role and that of other professionals with respect. It is probable the client recovers because of the total program and principally in interaction with his peers not because of any one person or discipline. As the counselor role becomes more structured, the counselor will develop a clearer sense of professional and personal identity. Ultimately, the counselor's "tool," like those of other mental health workers, consist of himself and the quality of the relationships he helps to create around him. The counselor's knowledge and skills will give him confidence, but his awareness of himself as a human being in the world will facilitate client recovery. He can help the client to explore himself only to the degree and depth that he has dared to explore his own inner self; he can assist the client to cope with outer realities to the extent he himself is aware of his environment.

Team work also demands that the counselor relinquish rescue fantasies and place the responsibility for recovery with the client. Alcohol compensates for unfilled essential needs. Consequently, the cure for the disease is a deep trust and involvement in living. No counselor or team, can provide these factors, although they can assist in the search and provide examples.

These attitudes in the counselor are very different from the peer-helping attitudes of the original AA counselors, who were recruited at Yale and elsewhere in 1940. Changing needs and changing systems have dictated other functions, and the role has become increasingly structured and specialized.

In common with other developing professions, credentialing has become an issue, and this will impact on training, and eventually, on the quality of care. The demand for credentialing of alcohol and drug counselors is linked to issues of limited public financing of alcoholism treatment and rehabilitation programs and the necessity of qualifying for third party payments. The insurance companies, in turn, must satisfy subscribers that certain standards of care are being met. Since it is not ordinarily possible for a purchaser of services either to judge quality or to shop and compare when under the pressure of an illness, public health and safety are at stake.

Credentialing allows for judgment of quality of services. It also serves as criteria for employment, standardization of care, and control of training, positions, and salaries. Historically, credentialing has meant a decrease of manpower, and an increase in costs. At issue are that these factors are balanced by an increase in quality care. The key elements in credentialing are knowledge, performance (competency), experience, and character (attitude). All these can be examined and discussed, but eventually someone must set standards.

In 1974, NIAAA contracted with Littlejohn Associates to study the credentialing of alcoholism counselors, focusing on three areas of need: assuring quality of care, obtaining third party payments, and public recognition of the counselor for their valuable services. The Littlejohn Report (1976), recommended the establishing of a national credentialing board. The NIAAA accepted the report but did not implement this suggestion for two reasons: a federal agency setting standards would seem to infringe on state rights, and HEW's moratorium on licensure activities, in order to slow the post-war proliferation of professions and specialties.

In spite of this, states were encouraged to set up their own credentialing procedures and may have done so. Most of these included requirements for experience in the field, as well as written and oral examinations.

As credentialing activity, however, became more widespread and, hence, more diverse, the need for national standards emerged even more clearly. In 1975, NIAAA responded to this need by establishing a Planning Panel under the chairmanship of Dr. Kenneth Finger. The final report of the Finger group, published in 1977, recommended that a National Credentialing Organization for

Alcoholism Counselors be established. Included would be a wide representation from the field. Moreover, it would be a self-supporting and independent professional group. The Federal government would provide initial start monies, but the organization would be self-supporting within five years. Preliminary activities to implement these findings are now underway.

The impact of the newly-trained counselors on their agency is another important stimulus for the upgrading of services and further demand for training. The newly-trained graduate comes back to his agency enthusiastic and ready to implement all he has learned. His enthusiasm and new ideas tend to stimulate other workers, which, in turn, raises functional expectations for all workers in the agency and generates a demand for new training.

With the gradually emerging role of the alcoholism counselor as a team worker having an inter-changeability of counseling functions with other professionals in the field of alcoholism treatment at the mid-level of expertise, it is doubtful if the term "paraprofessional" any longer applies. It needs to be stressed, however, that the alcoholism counselor, as other professionals, must be aware of the limitations of his discipline and call on others when the occasion warrants.

In common with the developmental history of other professions, we might predict ever-increasing demands for more highly trained and skilled workers. New knowledge, training, and certification will tend to raise the level of competence and thus, further structure and specialize the role. This, in turn, may tend to restrict new counselors from entering the field and ultimately raise the cost to employers and consumers.

Alcoholism service agencies had their beginning out of "store front" operations: they began as a peer response to a community need and tended to attract and serve the visible alcoholic—the deteriorated, chronic skid row type. With better funding for facilities, the trend has been to move away from "store front" operations, into facilities more attractive to middle class value systems. It is to be hoped that the better facilities will maintain the close and invaluable community contact of the early years of operation, when the agencies served those in greatest need.

In our own work with students, and close contact with the field over a 10-year period, we have been in a position to gather data and observe trends in the persons attracted to the field. In 1967, close to 70% of the counselors were male, white and between 40 and 45 years of age. The majority came from a vocational background of clerical, sales or "blue collar" jobs, almost 29% had a vocational background in the health or helping field and only 9 of 212 students were employed as alcoholism counselors prior to their enrollment in our training program. The majority had at least high school education, however, 3% had neither high school nor a General Education Diploma. On the other end of the scale, 30% had some college experience, 12% graduated at the baccalaureate level and 2% had an advanced degree. More than 50% of the counselors were recovering alcoholics.

In 1977, 10 years later, there were as many women as men in the profession. Their average age was between 31 and 42 years and their educational level much higher than in 1977; the number of counselors holding graduate degrees had doubled, and the percentage with some college experience had more than doubled. A total of 46.3% were recovering alcoholics. As for their vocational background, 72% of the counselors were previously employed in the human services field, and 70% had some specialized training in alcoholism.

One could conclude from the above figures that in the past 16 years, alcoholism counseling had moved from a vocation that attracted mid-level people with personal experience with the disease, into a specialty that increasingly attracted younger and better-educated human service workers. At present, the majority of alcoholism counselors have had some personal encounter with the effects of pathological drinking. They are either recovering alcoholics or have had personal contact with alcoholic relatives or "significant others." Another trend is now developing: workers from other fields, such as nursing, criminal justice, and welfare where the emotional rewards of successful client treatment have stimulated them to seek more knowledge and skills, seek to make alcoholism counseling a future specialty within their own profession.

## EVALUATION OF ALCOHOLISM COUNSELOR TRAINING PROGRAMS

Part of the evolution of alcoholism counseling—both as an independent role and as a set of skills within another profession—has involved the development of college- or university-based training programs. The utility and effectiveness of these programs is not always self-evident and requires appropriate evaluative instruments and methodologies. Since 1967, we have been involved with three training programs: Baltimore City Health Department Training Program for Alcoholism Counselors, Johns Hopkins University Continuing Education Program for Alcoholism Counselors, and the Regional Training Program for Alcoholism Counselors in Baltimore, Maryland. Some differences existed with respect to organization of the program and background of trainees. The Baltimore City program did not include an evaluation component until its final year (1974), while the Johns Hopkins and Regional Training programs had evaluation built in as a primary component. As one might expect, the instrumentation and methodology for the latter two programs were more complex and sophisticated. The content of the instruments—geared specifically to an alcoholism training program—are not relevant to a general volume on paraprofessionals. Our experience, however, allows us to make some general observations about the process of evaluating training programs.

The major lessons learned from the evaluation efforts carried out through this program were that: 1) data collection instruments need to be designed specifically for the program being evaluated, based on the curriculum of that program; and 2) the efforts needed to be consistent and comparable insofar as possible from class to class.

Evaluation is often the step-child of any program. As the central objective is to train (or treat, or otherwise serve) individuals, the continuous assessment of the program may seem a burdensome extravagance. However, our evaluation efforts have been used:

To assess the impact of the program on the trainee in terms of knowledge gained, opinion and effectiveness;

To refine and improve the training program; and

As the instruments for the testing of counselors for eventual credentialing.

Evaluation research is a dynamic discipline, particularly in the case of paraprofessional training and utilization. We must develop concepts and methods appropriate for use in this field instead of making futile attempts to force-fit concepts from other fields (e.g. basic research approaches of double-blind studies, strict control groups, etc.). The realities of both the training program, and the program in which the trainees will eventually work, must be considered. For example, Federal regulations regarding confidentiality of alcohol and drug abuse patient records, and the sensitive issue of patient's rights makes the impact of training on changes in the patient very difficult to assess. In addition, there have been few, if any, substantiated studies that can attribute changes in patient behavior to specific types of treatment, how can it be expected that one can accurately attribute—at two levels removed—training of a counselor or paraprofessional to changes in patient behavior? In fact, it is more reasonable to make the most defensible assessments of direct impact on the trainee, and indirectly on the program in which he/she is employed. If this impact has been positive and substantial, there is a highly positive outcome in itself.

The conduct of evaluation studies is often viewed by program administrators with skepticism. It is commonly recognized that many such studies carried out by external organizations have been valueless to the programs themselves; they, more often, serve the needs of a funding or review agency. Furthermore, those who are responsible for the evaluation tend not to render the results applicable to the programs themselves. When in-house evaluations are carried out, there may be a tendency for the evaluator to have vested interest in positive results, although if the design (including analytic procedure) is appropriate, it is difficult to adjust results to suit one's preferable outcome.

The evaluator, in house or external, bears a responsibility to develop appropriate designs and procedures that provide information that is both useful for the program, and insofar as possible reflective of the realities of program operation, taking into account exogenous variables as well as those directly related to the programs and their clients (trainees or patients). Evaluation need not be complex. Methods need to be developed that can be readily applied by program personnel, so that eventually the awe of, and often hostility toward, evaluation is replaced by an understanding of its usefulness for effective program operation.

## REFERENCES

Albee, G.W. *Mental health manpower trends*, New York: Basic Books, 1959.

Journal of AMA, October 20, 1916.

Littlejohn Corporation. Proposed National Standards for

Alcoholism Counselors. Report to National Institute of Alcohol Abuse and Alcoholism. Rockville, Md: 1976.

# III: PARAPROFESSIONALS: TRAINING, RESEARCH AND EVALUATION

# Evaluation of Paraprofessional Programs in the Human Services

Judith Blanton and Sam Alley,
*Social Action Research Center, Berkeley, California*


Any decision of whether to continue, expand, change, or terminate a paraprofessional program is a *de facto* evaluation. The question, therefore, is not whether to evaluate these programs but how systematically and meaningfully to do so; that is, whether to make these decisions on the basis of hunches, intuition or rumors, or with the aid of more systematically gathered and rigorously interpreted information. Pressures to develop more formal, sophisticated, and useful evaluations of paraprofessional programs seem to be increasing. These pressures are both external (requirements of funding sources and concerned citizens groups) and internal (from pro-

237

238 PARAPROFESSIONALS IN THE HUMAN SERVICES

gram administrators and staff who want better information with which to make decisions).

Despite strong pressures for evaluation, we have found few well-planned, well-implemented, and well-used evaluations in paraprofessional programs, even those with excellent reputations (Alley, Blanton, Feldman, Hunter, & Rolfson, Note 1). Indeed, evaluators are often welcomed to a program with slightly less enthusiasm than bearers of the bubonic plague.

### Why Are There Few Good Evaluations and Why Are Paraprofessional Programs Resistant to Doing Evaluations?

Most of the difficulties in doing good evaluations of paraprofessional programs are actually the same difficulties involved in doing good evaluations in general. The evaluation field is a young one. The sophistication of evaluation methods is increasing rapidly, however, and theories are clearly ahead of most current evaluation practice. There are also few well-trained evaluators. Only recently have graduate programs begun to offer courses in this area. Many people doing evaluation are self-taught and just "muddling through" without formal training. Costs are also an issue. Most paraprofessional programs are funded not as research projects but as action or service organizations. Thus, only a small proportion of resources is generally available for evaluation. Large, thorough evaluations are expensive, but if we want clear answers to some of the complex issues concerning paraprofessionals, we will have to allocate time, money, and effort to answer them. On the other hand, there are ways of making better use of evaluation activities within current budget limitations.

Although all of these issues are significant, they do not seem to account for the resistance to evaluations often voiced by service staff. The service staff of human services programs (including paraprofessional ones) complain that evaluators treat staff and clients as "things" rather than as people, and make unrealistic demands that hurt program operations. This includes such random selection of clients to receive some service, or demands that service staff keep extensive records. Service staff may feel used, rather than helped, by the evaluators, and may believe that evaluation efforts are an unnecessary diversion of resources that would be better spent on services. Wide gaps in status and salary between evaluators and service staff can also contribute to ill will.

Resistance to evaluations and, alternatively, pressure to evaluate are often political. The evaluator does not just supply information to add to the body of knowledge or to aid rational decision making. As Weiss (1975) describes, evaluation findings often become armaments for political battles, particularly around controversial and less established programs. Ironically, evaluations of well established programs are seldom done and seem to have little or no effect on their continuation.

The problems that paraprofessional programs are generally designed to combat (poverty, mental illness, crime, poor achievement, etc.) have complex and multiple causes. The evaluator's job is to determine the impact of the paraprofessional program from all the other factors. Moreover, when such multiple and complex factors operate, the paraprofessional program may be *necessary* but may not be *sufficient* to show any easily-measured impact on the problem.

Thus, from a social innovator's point of view, the typical evaluation of a budding or controversial program is inherently threatening and potentially destructive. In the battle for scarce resources, it may be more effective to argue the *need* for a particular paraprofessional program than to present the findings of an evaluation. As the Stanford Evaluation Consortium (1976) put it:

> Evaluators, in fact, can produce a strong case for
> withholding funds in the very instances where no
> such case could otherwise be mounted in the face of
> crushing social needs. In short, the reformers' an-
> tipathy to summative (i.e., outcome oriented) evalua-
> tion is not "paranoid" or "unthinking" or "anti-
> intellectual": it is simply pragmatic. (p.201)

Finally, one of the major sources of resistance to evaluating paraprofessional programs has been the mystique surrounding paraprofessionals themselves. The
commitment to paraprofessional education and training
has often been ideological. A mystique has often sur-
rounded these programs that has made the very notion of
evaluation seem not only unnecessary but even base or
the tool of reactionary destroyers. In such an atmosphere,
evaluators must take special pains to assure service staff
members that critical reflection about activities is not
traitorous, but potentially constructive. The concept of
the "loyal opposition," which has served parliamentary
government, might be useful as a stance for evaluators
who are working with staffs possessing strong ideological
commitments.

## WHAT CAN BE DONE TO IMPROVE EVALUATION OF PARAPROFESSIONAL PROGRAMS?

What can be done to make evaluations useful, to have
them aid, rather than hinder, social innovation? How can
service staffs become more cooperative in studying their
program and more open to evaluation findings? This article will attempt to deal with these questions by describing
five areas in which paraprofessional programs are generally evaluated, the typical model of evaluation, and an
alternative model. We will deal with issues such as the
use of evaluation as a part of the planning process, determining what to assess, evaluation as intervention,

evaluation of developing projects, evaluation as a developmental process, and strategies for integrating evaluation findings.

The basic evaluation question in paraprofessional programs is: What kinds of paraprofessionals can do what kinds of tasks with what degree of effectiveness given what kind of training, education, supportive services and supervision on the job? (Grant and Grant, 1975)

In general, evaluations of paraprofessional programs can be grouped into six general areas.

1. *Evaluations of the effects of paraprofessional programs in improving services to individual clients and the community.* Evaluations of this type focus on the quality and quantity of services delivered by paraprofessionals. Gartner (Note 2) reviews the literature on the effectiveness of paraprofessionals in mental health. Carkhuff (1968) compares lay and professional wages.

2. *Education and training.* Evaluation of education and training programs tends to focus on the effectiveness of the implementation of education and/or training programs for paraprofessionals. Some of the evaluations examine the effect of the training on the paraprofessional (increase in skill, changes in attitude, etc.), and occasionally such evaluations consider the impact of the training on improvement of services. D'Augelli (Note 3), Truax (1965), and some of our work (Alley, Blanton, Churgin, and Grant, 1973; Alley, Blanton, Churgin, and Grant, 1974) provide examples of this.

3. *Job and career development evaluations.* During the late 1960s, many paraprofessional programs had as a primary goal the employment of poor, indigenous populations. New Careers goals included the development of *careers* rather than dead end, "soft money", jobs. New Careers philosophy urged the creation of meaningful and hu-

manly useful jobs for individuals who had previously been denied access to the opportunity structure. More recently, attention has shifted to possibilities for horizontal and vertical mobility for paraprofessional workers within the system. The work of Gartner, Riessman, and Jackson (1977) and of Alley et al. (1974) examine these issues.

4. *Organization and systems change.* Evaluations in this area assess the extent to which paraprofessional employees changed the organization or community where they were employed. Examples are making the organization more responsive to the community, changing the patterns of services delivered, changing the roles of professionals within the organization, and changing relations between professionals and paraprofessionals. Sobey (1970), Delworth (1974), and Alley and Blanton (1974) look at these issues, but clearly more work in this area is needed.

5. *Descriptions of and changes in the paraprofessionals themselves.* Evaluations of this type describe kinds of people working in paraprofessional programs. Such studies may describe kinds of paraprofessionals more likely to complete training, receive promotions, or drop out. Other evaluations in this area asses changes in the paraprofessionals' skills, values, roles, sues, roles, self-concept, etc., as a result of their education, training, and/or work. See Kelleher, Kerr, and Melville (1968), McClelland and Rhodes (1969), and Gartner, Costa, Gillooly, and Gross (1975).

6. *Economic effectiveness.* Although one of the major arguments for the use of paraprofessional staff is their cost effectiveness, surprisingly little serious study has been made of this issue. Conant (1973) and Marschak and Henke (Note 4) provide suggestions about how to evaluate this area.

Not only are the areas that are evaluated quite diverse, but so are the methodologies and even the purposes of evaluations. A look at the *Handbook of Evaluation Research* (Struening and Guttentag, 1975) shows the lack of agreement among the leaders in the field. Different kinds of evaluation imply different criteria for judging a "good" evaluation and different, often contradictory, research tactics.

The authors will describe what they see as the dominant model in the evaluation of paraprofessional programs and then describe what we see as an alternative model.

Typically, paraprofessional evaluations are commissioned by the funding agency. They generally begin after the program has been planned or even implemented. The evaluator, or evaluators, may be hired from outside as consultants or subcontractors, or, alternatively, be part of the internal staff of the agency. Evaluation activities run parallel to other program operations. The evaluators make observations and collect information but generally do not have much interaction with service staff. The process ends abruptly with a formal, written report to a decision maker.

An alternative model for evaluating paraprofessional programs is based largely on our own experience as evaluators of paraprofessional programs, but it is quite similar to the model proposed by the Stanford Evaluation Consortium (1976) in their critique of the *Handbook of Evaluation Research* (Struening and Guttentag, 1975).

Our alternative model is based on a number of guiding principles.

1.  Evaluation can, and should, be used as part of the planning process.
2.  Evaluation should be an integral and ongoing part of the program design, not just tacked on to meet outside demands.
3.  The evaluator can, and should, be a tool to improve

program quality and to assist program staff to be more aware of what they are doing, how they are doing it, and what they are achieving.

4. The evaluation can, itself, be a development process. The evaluator need not limit concerns to objectives stated in advance, but can function as a naturalistic observer whose inquiries grow out of observations.

5. The consumers of evaluation findings should have a clear understanding of what the evaluation involves, and findings should be fed back to them in usable form as early as possible.

6. The integration of findings into program decision making does not happen automatically, and efforts to integrate findings must take into account resistance to the findings.

The rest of this article will examine a number of issues that will elaborate on this alternative model and give examples of how to apply this model to evaluations of paraprofessional programs. These issues include the use of evaluation as a part of the planning process, problems in assessing what to assess, difficulties in evaluating developing projects, looking at evaluation itself as a developmental process, and how to integrate evaluation feedback.[1]

## EVALUATION AS A PART OF PLANNING

Building in the evaluation from the beginning of program planning and operations makes the evaluation

[1] A discussion of statistical and technical methodologies which could be used in paraprofessional evaluation strategies would be too lengthy to pursue here, so we will refer the reader to a list of references included at the end of this paper, which the authors hope will help the interested reader design methods appropriate for the problem to be studied.

more effective as well as more readily carried out. Having data collection requirements spelled out from the start and included (if appropriate) in job descriptions reduces resistance from service staff who generally object when suddenly asked to add evaluation activities to an already busy schedule. Designing the evaluation before the program begins makes it easier to build in evaluation instruments and set up control groups or any other structures that might be necessary for the evaluation design.

Yet, the primary argument for beginning evaluation activities early is not for the sake of the *evaluation* but for the sake of the program. Activities such as needs assessment, goal setting, clarification of objectives, determining how alternative strategies can be expected to lead to goal accomplishment, and setting up expected time frames by which objectives should be reached, are not just evaluation activities but useful parts of the planning process.

## DETERMINING WHAT TO ASSESS: THE CASE OF GOALS

Texts on evaluation generally focus on methodologies that can be used to measure a goal. Although some attention is given on how to convert a broad, abstract goal into a measurable objective, there is seldom any attention given to the problem of deciding exactly what is the program's goal. In our first evaluations of paraprofessional programs, we naïvely assumed that the goals of the program were those written in the proposal, but when we began to look more closely at what the paraprofessional programs were doing, we found it was seldom that simple.

Many paraprofessional programs were developed with federal funding (Title I of ESEA, Career Opportunity Programs of the Office of Education, New Careers Programs of the Department of Labor, or Paraprofessional Manpower Programs of NIMH). The federal agencies administering these programs set goals that projects had to espouse (at least on paper) so that they could obtain funding. In most cases, the local programs embraced the federal goals but had their own goals as well, goals which sometimes took priority over federal goals.

Attention to stated goals is generally not enough. It is important to look at the unintended consequences, both positive and negative, of paraprofessional programs. For example, we have noted unintended consequences of paraprofessional programs to include such positive benefits as increased personal growth of the paraprofessionals, more sensitivity of an agency to client needs, and such negative results as increased stress within the families of the paraprofessionals or increased frustration if training programs did not lead to permanent jobs.

Discussions about goals at the early stages of project planning or operation also assist project staff in clarifying what they want to do. Project activities should be strategies designed to meet goals. Too often, however, the process happens backward. A group of people know how to do something (train staff) or decide that something would be good to do (hire indigenous community people) and, thus, are invested in the project activities (strategies). They, then, look for community needs or goals that would justify and support these strategies. In some instances, the relationship among stated community needs, program goals, and program activities is never firmly made. There will be goals stated but no program activities specifically developed to meet these goals. Alternatively, there will be a substantial amount of resources allocated to certain program activities that do not clearly relate to any of the stated program goals.

The discussions of program goals should include clarification of what the project is doing to meet those goals. If there are program activities that are not linked to program goals, does this indicate there are additional implicit goals to be stated? The authors worked with one project which had written goals including developing career ladders for their paraprofessionals. When the authors looked at their allocation of resources, we found that virtually all funds were spent on the *training* of the paraprofessional staff. No staff member was clearly designated to work on developing career ladders or knowledgeable in this area although she/he had been given the assignment. The evaluation, concerned with goals and the strategies to reach those goals, led to the director's decision to reallocate resources, hire an individual with skills in job analysis, and developing of career ladders.

## EVALUATION AS INTERVENTION

In all evaluation models, there is general agreement that evaluation *findings* constitute an intervention into the program operations. We take a more radical stand believing that the *decision to do* a formal evaluation, the *planning* of the evaluation, and the evaluation *implementation* all affect program operations. Further, we believe that evaluations can be designed in such a way as to be a positive intervention which improves program quality. Some of the examples we have cited previously indicate ways in which the process of evaluation can be used to improve program planning and resource evaluation. The famous Hawthorne studies (Parsons, 1974) vividly describe how attempts to measure can actually affect the thing the researcher is attempting to measure. An evaluator of paraprofessional programs needs to learn from these studies in two ways. First, in designing measurement tools, the evaluator seeking the most valid and reliable information should try to avoid "reactive" measures. In their now classic book, *Unobtrusive Measures: Nonreactive Research in the Social Sciences* (Webb, Campbell, Schwartz, and Sechrest, 1966), the authors provide a number of useful ideas on how to design and use measures that minimize obtrusive effects of the measurement tools themselves. A beneficial side effect of using unobtrusive measures is that they are often less costly than elaborate measurement batteries.

The Hawthorne studies also suggest ways that evaluation interventions can be used positively. For example, an evaluation design that elicits input from clients and service staff and uses this information to affect program policy should increase the morale of these groups since it actually increases their power and sense of efficacy. Questions aimed at program administrators can draw their attention to areas they may have neglected, and these questions can subtly suggest they should devote more effort to these areas. Meetings to clarify goal statements can increase group agreement about program purposes and increase group cohesion and efficiency. Evaluation interventions can also be used positively if problem-oriented reviews of program activities uncover problems before they reach crisis proportions. Highly judgmental, punitive evaluations, on the other hand, result in a tendency to hide problems and to blame others, and thus reduce capacity for constructive problem solving.

If the evaluation becomes part of the intervention, it is necessary to study the evaluation as well. An interesting and neglected area of research is the positive and negative impact of different kinds of evaluations on staff function, program functioning, and service impact.

What are the general implications for paraprofessional programs of understanding that evaluation can be an intervention? For projects which are primarily interested in improving their own functions rather than generalizing from their results, evaluation strategies can be used to enhance program planning, decision making, and group awareness about program purposes. In those projects interested in generalizing beyond a specific setting to contribute to the research base about paraprofessional programs in general, it may be necessary to add the impact of evaluation as a formal independent variable whose impact on program functioning is examined. If an evaluation process has a major impact within a program, then generalizations about the utility of that program model would need to include recognition that evaluation processes form an integral part of the program model.

## DESIGNING EVALUATIONS FOR DEVELOPING PROJECTS

In evaluating paraprofessional programs in the human services, we believe it is important to design evaluations which take into account the fact creating such programs is a developmental process. Rather than springing full blown as Athena from Zeus's head, most paraprofessional programs must go through a period of parturition and growing pains before reaching maturity. Too often, we do not take into account that beginning a program and building a staff are themselves important developmental tasks which must be dealt with before the program can effectively service clients.

Both funding agencies and programs, themselves, must recognize that staff building, planning, and start-up time are necessary to the development of a strong project. If project funders do not recognize this, they may ignore programs that may be desperately needed and potentially effective but are not highly sophisticated. Similarly, funders may cut off funding to a program that has the potential for providing an important and useful service but is having problems in its early phases. Ironically, if the *need* for such a program is clear, a similar program may be funded in the same community soon after the demise of the old one, but it will have to begin all over again. In terms of costs and benefits, it could be better to continue to support struggling programs if they show clear signs of developmental progress. Longer funding periods and evaluations that looked at process as well as outcomes could help in this process.

Pressures on the paraprofessional projects for quick progress may result in the project's staff making exaggerated claims for what they will accomplish during the first year. Project staff may react by moving into full scale operations without sufficient planning. If they find goals difficult to meet, they may react by hiding, rather than dealing with, problems and losing morale.

A project's relation with other agencies may also be affected by the kind of evaluation planned. For example, in a program using paraprofessionals to work with delinquent youth, other agencies (schools, probation and police) were reluctant to refer youth to the program because they knew the program had only short term funding and faced a stringent outcome evaluation. In the words of one probation officer, "I don't want to refer a kid and then have the program collapse." Ironically, the lack of referrals was a primary cause of the program's poor evaluation. Thus, a good evaluation should assist the project in setting realistic goals. These may need to be negotiated with the funding agent to maintain high standards but allow high risk programs the chance to establish themselves.

## EVALUATION AS A DEVELOPMENTAL PROCESS

Traditional models of evaluation are "pseudo-experimental" (Edwards, Guttentag, & Snapper, 1975) ones in which the evaluator insists that the program stay motionless while the evaluator takes a picture of it. Paraprofessional projects operate in what Emery and Trist (1972) call the "turbulent setting." Such projects often change in focus or direction. The kinds of paraprofessionals employed or trained may change or the kinds of jobs in which they work may shift.

Although the authors believe it is necessary to start an evaluation with some clear, well-thought-out plan, they also contend that evaluations, themselves, should be viewed as developmental. Periodic reviews of the evaluation design and of the status of the program can be used to determine if the evaluation is assessing the areas that are of most importance. If it is found that the evaluation is ignoring important issues or focusing on areas that are no longer of significance, modifications in the evaluation instruments or design could be considered. Caution, of course, is required. The potential benefits of any change must be weighed against the effort required to change and any loss of existing information. Pilot testing of instruments and soliciting feedback from respondants can be very helpful in determining if crucial areas were tapped or ignored or if confusion in interpretation of items or instructions was experienced.

## INTEGRATION OF FINDINGS

Too often, paraprofessional projects are evaluated and the findings are never used to improve program operations. In clinical practice the authors are well aware of the inadequacy of just telling someone what is wrong and suggesting ways of correcting those problems; however, many researchers continue to do just this in most program evaluations. Integration of evaluation findings is an important process that can not be taken for granted (Weiss, 1973). Although the authors have discussed methods for integrating findings back into decision making elsewhere (Blanton and Alley, Note 5) the following strategies should be mentioned here.

1. More involvement of evaluation consumers in the findings can increase the probability that the findings will be accepted and integrated into decision making. The best strategy for making consumers of evaluation *feel* involved is to *involve* them in the planning and operation of the evaluation and in the interpretation of the impact of findings. An attempt should be made to avoid a polarization between evaluation and service staff

and to create a climate of trust and mutual helpfulness.

2.  Pacing the findings is important. Information should be available in time to make crucial decisions, not after the decisions have been made.

3.  Integration of findings is helped by avoiding technical, jargon laden, unwieldy reports. A good format includes a clear, short, readable summary; a list of major findings; and implications and recommendations. Visual displays and simple charts can also be helpful.

4.  If there are a number of audiences for the evaluation findings, short summary reports can be prepared which emphasize data and implications relevant to the interests of each group. The complete report may be too cumbersome for groups to find the answers to their particular questions quickly and easily.

5.  It is useful to supplement written evaluation findings with dissemination of results through workshops or discussions with key groups.

6.  We have found project staff to be more receptive to reports of problems when what the program is doing right is also mentioned.

7.  There are generally several ways to interpret findings (numbers don't speak for themselves). Alternative explanations for findings should be presented along with any anecdotal or case study material that could suggest which interpretation is most likely.

8.  Besides describing what the program accomplished, the evaluator interested in influencing policy might explore "what plausible further directions of program development might appeal to various segments of the decision-making community and to make predictions about those alternative models on the basis of his accumulated

knowledge." (Stanford Evaluation Consortium, 1976.

More attention needs to be given to the quality of evaluations in paraprofessional programs. Improving the evaluation of paraprofessional programs is a key strategy to improving the quality of the programs themselves. Evaluations can provide information on how effectively program activities are progressing (process evaluation), the extent to which goals and objectives are met (outcome evaluation), and whether community needs are ultimately served by the project (evaluation of relevance).

A variety of different types of evaluation designs and methods are required to suit a variety of programs and policy needs. Staff of paraprofessional programs and their funding agents must be careful to select the kind of evaluation that will provide information necessary to answer their specific questions. The authors believe that paraprofessional programs today need to move beyond evaluation models which only give *post hoc* judgments to ones providing a program with ongoing information that can improve its operations.

## REFERENCE NOTES

1. D'Augelli, A. R. *Strategies for the comprehensive evaluation of training programs for nonprofessional human service workers.* Paper presented at the American Psychological Association Convention, Montreal, August 1973.

## REFERENCES

Alley, S., & Blanton, J. *Service delivery in new careers projects.* Berkeley, Calif: Social Action Research Center, 1974.

Alley, S., Blanton, J., & Churgin, S. *New careers programs in community mental health: Variables and models*: Berkeley, Calif.: Social Action Research Center, 1974.

Alley, S., Blanton, J., Churgin, S., and Grant, J.D. *Strategies for change in mental health; new careers* (4 Vols.). Berkeley, Calif.: Social Action Research Center, 1973.

Alley, S., Blanton, J., Churgin, S., & Grant, J.D. *New Careers: Strategies for change in mental health* (3 Vols.). Berkeley, Calif.: Social Action Research Center, 1974.

Alley, S. R., Blanton, J., Feldman, R. E., Hunter, G. D., & Rolfson, M. *Paraprofessionals in mental health; Twelve effective programs*. New York, N.Y.: Human Sciences Press, 1979.

Blanton, J., & Alley, S. How evaluation findings can be integrated into program decision making. *Community Mental Health Journal*, 1978, 14(3), 239-247.

Carkhuff, R. R. Differential functioning of lay and professional helpers. *Journal of Counseling Psychology*, 1968, *15*, 117-126.

Conant, E. H. *Teacher and Paraprofessional Work Productivity: A Public School Cost Effectiveness Study*. Lexington, Mass.: Lexington Books, 1973.

Delworth, U.A. Paraprofessionals as guerillas: Recommendations for systems change. *Personnel and Guidance Journal*, 1974, *53*, 335-338

Edwards, W., Guttentag, M., & Snapper, K. A decision-theoretic approach to evaluation research. In E. L. Streuning & M. Guttentag (Eds.), *Handbook of Evaluation Research* (Vol. 1). Beverly Hills, Calif.: Sage Publications, 1975.

Emery, F. E., & Trist, E. L. The causal texture of organizational environments. In F. E. Emery (Ed.), *Systems Thinking*. Baltimore, Md.: Penguin Books, 1972.

Gartner, A., Costa., Gillooly, F., & Gross, I. *A Comparative study of career opportunities program graduates as first-year teachers*. New York: New Careers Training Laboratory, 1975.

Gartner, A. The effectiveness of paraprofessionals in service delivery. In S. R. Alley, J. Blanton, & R. E. Feldman (Eds.), *Paraprofessionals in mental health: Theory and practice*. New York, N.Y.: Human Sciences Press, 1979.

Gartner, A., F. Riessman, & V. C. Jackson. *Paraprofessionals in education today. New York: Human Sciences Press, 1977.*

Grant, J., & Grant, J.D. Evaluation of new careers programs. In M. Guttentag & E. L. Struening (Eds.), *Handbook of Evaluation Research* (Vol.2). Beverly Hills, Calif.: Sage Publications, 1975.

Kelleher, E. J., Kerr, W. A., & Melville, N. T. The prediction of subprofessional nursing success. *Personnel Psychology*, 1968, *21*, 379-388.

Marschak, T., & Henke, C. Achieving economic efficiency with paraprofessionals. In S. R. Alley, J. Blanton, & R. E. Feldman (Eds.), *Paraprofessionals in mental health: Theory and practice*. New York, NY, Human Sciences Press, 1979

McClelland, J.N., & Rhodes, F. Prediction of job success for hospital aides and orderlies from MMPI scores and personal history data. *Journal of Applied Psychology*, 1969, *53*, 49-54.

Parsons, H. M. What happened at Hawthorne? *Science*, 1974, *183*, 922-932.

Sobey, F. *The Nonprofessional revolution in mental health*. New York: Columbia University Press, 1970.

Stanford Evaluation Consortium. Evaluating the handbook of evaluation research. In G. V. Glass (Ed.), *Evaluation Studies Review Annual* (Vol.1). Beverly Hills, Calif.: Sage Publications, 1976.

Struening, E. L., & Guttentag, M. (Eds.), *Handbook of evaluation research* (Vol. 1). Beverly Hills, Calif.: Sage Publications, 1975.

Truax, C. B. *An approach to training for the aid therapist: Research and implications.* Fayetteville, Ark.: Arkansas Rehabilitation Research and Training Center, 1965.

Webb. E. J., Campbell, D. T., Schwartz, R. D., & Sechrest, L. *Unobtrusive measures: Nonreactive research in the social sciences.* Chicago: Rand McNally College Publishing Co., 1966.

Weiss, C.H. Between the cup and the lip. *Evaluation,* 1973, *1,* 159-165.

Weiss. C. H. Evaluation research in the political context. In E. L. Struening & M. Guttentag (Eds.), *Handbook of evaluation research* (Vol. 1). Beverly Hills, Calif.: Sage Publications, 1975.

## ADDITIONAL READINGS IN STATISTICAL METHODOLOGIES

Bloom, B. Mental health program evaluation. In S. E. Golann & C. Eisdorfer (Eds.), *Handbook of community mental health.* New York: Appleton-Century-Crofts, 1972.

Campbell, D. Reforms as experiments. In C. H. Weiss (Ed.), *Evaluating action programs.* Boston: Allyn & Bacon, 1972.

Campbell, D. T., & Stanley, J. C. *Experimental and quasi-experimental designs for research.* Chicago: Rand McNally, 1963.

Hargreaves, W. A., Atkisson, C. C., Siegel, L. M., & McIntyre, M. H. (Eds.). *Resource materials for community mental health program evaluation. Part IV—Evaluating the effectiveness of services* (DHEW Publication No. [ADM] 75-222). Rockville, Md.: National Institute of Mental Health, 1975.

Mager, R. F. *Goal analysis.* Belmont, Ca.: Fearon Publishers, 1972.

Rossi, P.H. Testing for success and failure in social action.

In P.H. Rossi & W. Willians (Eds.), *Evaluating social programs*. New York: Seminar Press, 1972.

Suchman, E. A. Action for what? A critique of evaluative research. In C. H. Weiss (Ed.), *Evaluating action programs: Readings of social action and education*. Boston: Allyn and Bacon, 1972.

Suchman, E. A. *Evaluative research: Principles and practice in public research*. New York: Russell Sage, 1967.

Weiss, C. H. *Evaluation Research: Methods of assessing program effectiveness*. Englewood Cliffs, N.J.: Prentice-Hall, 1972.

# Parapro's and Paraprose:
# The Case of the Paraprofessional in the
# Community Mental Health Center

William J. Riley,
*Department of Hospital and Health Care
Administration
School of Public Health,
University of Minnesota,*


Morton O. Wagenfeld and Stanley S. Robin,
*Department of Sociology,
Western Michigan University*

In this chapter a controversial issue prominent in community mental health will be examined: the paraprofessional worker in the community mental health center. It is fairly well accepted that the sociopolitical climate of ameliorative optimism of the early 1960s influenced the development of both the community mental health and paraprofessional movement (Robin and Wagenfeld, 1976). Concerns about "ethnic power," the war on poverty, and racism were important factors in the genesis of both phenomena. Part of the inherent importance of community mental health has been its capacity to fill a previously unmet need to serve those who had been denied, or given only the most rudimentary mental health care (e.g., Geiger, 1967; Riessman, 1963; Robin and Wagenfeld, 1977). Much of the appeal of, and support for, the use of paraprofessionals has been to serve those who have been given little or insufficient human services as well as providing employment for those who have been given little occupational opportunity.

## Genesis of the Paraprofessional in the CMHC

Their history reveals that the paraprofessional in community mental health did not arrive at that destination by design. Rather, through a convergence of several forces, a niche arose in the Community Mental Health Center (CMHC) and the paraprofessional became an acquired member of the treatment team. Since the inception of the CMHC movement, one of the most critical problems has been the lack of trained manpower to to provide care and treatment (Littlestone, 1964; David, 1969). In the early planning stages, numerous committees and commissions assessed the manpower shortage confronting the CMHCs (e.g., Joint Commission on Mental Illness and Health, 1961; McKnickle and Higman, 1964). There was never any serious consideration, however, given to employing the indigenous poor (for example, see Albee, 1959). Full understanding of how the concept of the paraprofessional worker was conceived requires examination of a parallel social movement. In 1964 Congress initiated an innovative program to eradicate poverty in the United States. This legislation was entitled the Economic Opportunity Act and it established the Office of Economic Opportunity (OEO). The Economic Opportunity Act not only proposed to help the poor help themselves, it also demanded that there be a "maximum feasible participation" of the poor (Title II). At about the same time, a novel phrase "new careers" appeared in the title of a book written by Pearl and Riessman (1965). *New Careers for the Poor* advocated the use of nonprofessionals in human services. The interest was in eliminating the "unforgivable shame of poverty" but the novelty of their idea was to use the position of the paraprofessional in the training of the indigenous poor for a career. This training would subsequently enable the trainee to climb out of poverty. For the purpose of this analysis, it is crucial to point out that the employment of paraprofessionals in a career ladder was a strategy developed to help the poor, not to help the CMHC, since in their work, Pearl and Riessman had no particular interest in the CMHC movement. As the paraprofessionals became entrenched in the CMHC, however, a more sophisticated rationale emerged and assertions were made that the paraprofessionals could relate to the client more effectively than the professional (Torrey, 1969) because they have a special sensitivity and compassion with clients by nature of their common poverty background (Arnhoff et al., 1969b).

Concern began to be expressed that the paraprofessionals were becoming co-opted by the CMHC professionals (Haug and Sussman, 1969). It was charged that a "manipulation of access" occurred among those selected for employment and Ritzer (1974) contended that this constituted co-optation. It was also maintained that the paraprofessionals could be considered co-opted if they lost their identity with the community. For example, as the result of training, Christmas (1966) concluded that the behavior change of paraprofessionals was "most striking." Most important, these changes appeared to be in the direction of the "status quo" (Miller, et al., 1970).

There existed, nevertheless, indications to the professionals that strong activism would accompany the introduction of paraprofessionals into community health agencies (e.g., Minuchin, 1969; Ahearn, 1970). Paraprofessionals were referred to as activists because they were truly concerned about the services rendered to "their own people" (Boyette, 1971). On the other hand, it was also feared that they might uncover "explosive social problems" (Willcox, 1970) and "assert power" (Albrecht, 1974).

## THE PARAPROFESSIONAL IN THE CMHC: THE FOCUS OF THE RESEARCH[1]

The authors intend to examine evidence regarding the issues of co-optation and activism among paraprofessionals employed in CMHCs. Moreover, they will explore the degree to which activism exists among paraprofessionals by examining their roles in CMHCs. Role is conceptualized in three ways: *CMHC role activism* is the measurement of activism in the role of the community mental health worker from the worker's perspective of his Center's expectations. *Personal/Professional role activism* is the measurement of activism in the role of community mental health worker from the perspective of the preferred behaviors of the worker—free of organizational constraints. *Role discrepancy* is the difference between

[1]This paper is part of a larger study. Descriptions of rationale, instrumentation and methods can be found elsewhere (cf. Robin and Wagenfeld, 1976, 1977; Wagenfeld and Robin, 1976). An extended discussion of the development of the paraprofessional movement in general, and the paraprofessional in the community mental health center, in particular, can be found in, Riley, W. The paraprofessional polemic: Investigating the case of the paraprofessional in the community mental health center. M.A. thesis, Western Michigan University, 1976.

these scores calculated for each worker. It can be viewed as an index of a kind of role conflict in assuming the community mental health worker role.

The absolute amount of CMHC activism included in the role by the paraprofessionals and its comparison with the CMHC activism of the professionals provides an insight into the socialization of the paraprofessional to the CMHC in which he or she is employed. If one of the reasons for introducing paraprofessionals into CMHCs was to inculcate a degree of indigenous social activism in the organization, then the magnitude and direction of CMHC activism is an index of the nature and effect of paraprofessionals in CMHCs. Three logical possibilities exist in the interpretation of CMHC activism findings. If the paraprofessionals are high and the professionals low in CMHC activism, then one may infer that the paraprofessionals are bringing an increased level of activism to their centers. If the paraprofessional and the professional are high in CMHC activism, then one can infer that either the paraprofessionals have been successful in the infusion of activism into their organizations or that activism was present in the Centers independent of the paraprofessionals. If the two groups are both low in CMHC activism, then it can be inferred that the paraprofessionals were co-opted or that the expectation that paraprofessionals would be purveyors of activism was in error.

Personal/professional activism yields a more direct measure of paraprofessional socialization and co-optation. Following the logic employed in the preceding paragraph, if the paraprofessionals are high and the professionals low in personal/professional activism, then it would appear that the paraprofessionals are different and have not been co-opted in their perspective. If the paraprofessionals and the professionals are both high in personal/professional activism, then one can infer that while the paraprofessionals have not been co-opted, they have not added a unique perspective, *vis-à-vis* activism, to the potential behavior in providing community mental health services. If both groups are low in personal/professional activism: then one can infer that the paraprofessionals have been co-opted in their perspective on the role or that they were inappropriate for adding a unique perspective to the potential behavior in providing community mental health services. A fourth possibility exists for both CMHC and personal professional activism: the paraprofessionals are low in activism and the professionals are high. If this is the case, both the nature of the problem and its solution has been misconstrued in the literature.

Role discrepancy, the difference between the two forms of activism, gives insight into the nature and effects of co-optation. If the paraprofessionals manifest low role discrepancy as a result of a low CMHC activism and low personal/professional activism, then co-optation can be seen as an adjustive mechanism of the paraprofessional in his/her role. Alternatively, it can mean that the activism expectations held for the paraprofessionals are erroneous. If low role discrepancy is a result of high CMHC and personal/professional activism, then the paraprofessional has achieved a role adjustment by perceiving the center's definition of his/her role with the same high level of activism as he/she brings to the personal/professional role definition. The validity of this role adjustment can be verified by noting the level of CMHC activism by the professionals. High role discrepancy for the paraprofessional as a consequence of low CMHC activism and high personal/professional activism would indicate a state of tension among the paraprofessionals that, conceivably, could make the role of the paraprofessional difficult to maintain and their viability in the center problematic. This situation, however, would indicate that one of the predictions attending the creation of the paraprofessional—greater activism in the center—was tenable.

In order to understand the experiences and characteristics of the paraprofessional, and whether they bring a new element to the community mental health worker (CMHW) role, several variables were examined for their relationship to the paraprofessional role definition of CMHW. Broadly, the authors believed that four categories of variables would have important predictive influence on role activism, and discrepancy: personal characteristics of the paraprofessionals, type of center participation, characteristics of the CMHC's catchment area, and organizational characteristics of the CMHCs. More specifically, the personal characteristics were: age, sex, level of education, and endorsement of the ideology of community mental health. Type of center participation included years at center and time spent in direct and indirect services. The nature of the CMHC's catchment area was defined in terms of socioeconomic status, ethnicity and geographic complexity (degree of urbanization). Finally, the last set of factors—structural characteristics of the CMHC—was operationalized as: auspices, organizational complexity, and locus of accountability. (For a more extended discussion of these factors see Riley, 1976.)

## METHOD

As indicated earlier, this research is part of a larger study. The objective of the larger study was an examination of the degree of activism in the role of community mental health workers. Community mental health workers were defined as professional and paraprofessional staff employed by CMHCs.[2] In order to obtain a sample of workers, 20 CMHCs were selected for the research as representative of the major catchment area and organiza-

[2] A roster of CMHC staff and their position were obtained from each center. Job title, professional affiliation, education, and other personal data were self-reported. Anomalies in the classification of workers were resolved by contact with center director and his/her staff.

tional characteristics of operating centers.[3]

Indices were developed to measure the catchment area characteristics of: socio-economic status, ethnicity and demographic complexity (Wagenfeld, et al., 1974). A total of three organizational characteristics of CMHCs were delineated: organizational complexity, auspices, and accountability (Wagenfeld, et al., 1974).

The dependent variables were measured through the development of The Community Mental Health Worker Role Inventory (CMHWRI). The CMHWRI consisted of a series of 18 vignettes. Each vignette represented a community situation that a worker might encounter. A total of nine areas of community life were represented. The workers were asked to select the appropriate behaviors from a series of possible behaviors that ranged from exclusion (the vignette calling for some community action was excluded as not proper for the CMHW role) to highly activist (the selection of behaviors to change the community by collective action outside of established community structures).

The concept of co-optation was defined as the paraprofessionals' absorption of the goals, values, and expectations of the CMHC in preference to the expectations of the client or community. Activism was defined as the willingness of the paraprofessionals to violate the expec-

[3]Mailed questionnaires were sent to all staff in accordance with methods developed by Glock and Stark (1966) and Robin (1965). A 56% response rate was obtained (N-595) of whom 95 were identified as paraprofessionals. Analysis of non-respondents by occupational affiliation did not reveal any large-scale anomalies for the professionals. The paraprofessionals, however, had the lowest response rate of any occupational category (34%). Subsequent analysis on the paraprofessionals indicated that non-respondents tended to come disproportionately from those with low education and were more likely to be younger and male. These qualifications should be borne in mind when interpreting the data. Additional data, however, not reported here (Riley, 1976) indicate that the non-respondents among the paraprofessionals are *more conservative* than those who did respond. This response bias would likely accentuate differences between the paraprofessionals and professionals.

tations of the community mental health center so that the needs of the community or client could be served.

## FINDINGS

A logical first step is a two-fold examination of the measures of role activism and role discrepancy. Our data suggest that CMHC and personal/professional activism —as we have measured them—are not strongly held by either professional or paraprofessional workers. Both groups are found concentrated in the lower ranges of the scores. Only the personal/professional activism score of professionals is in the third quartile, and, as indicated by cumulative scores, less than one percent of them do so.

The data on role discrepancy indicate that it is not found at a high level in either paraprofessionals or professionals: virtually all respondents in both groups score within the first quartile. Further, there are no significant differences between the paraprofessionals and the rest of the CMHC staff on any of the role measurements.

At this juncture, one might infer that if paraprofessionals were brought into CMHCs in an effort to inject a note of community activism. This does not appear to have happened. They are virtually identical to other staff. The authors noted in an earlier section, however, that a similarity of scores might be compatible with several explanations. This point will be considered further in the following sections.

Having noted that the paraprofessionals do not differ from their professional colleagues in activism or discrepancy, the authors have to introduce a qualification. To present the professionals as a single group as a counterpose to paraprofessionals is to fail to recognize the heterogeneous character of the former and perhaps mask some significant differences.

In comparing paraprofessionals to each of the major occupational groups in the CMHCs, the authors found that no significant differences existed in perception of CMHC role.

Table 1

Paraprofessional and Other Workers Personal/Professional Role Activism Scores[*]

| Worker Affiliation | N | X[+] | SD | t test between parapro- fessionals and each group of workers | P (one tail) |
|---|---|---|---|---|---|
| Psychiatrists | 72 | 40.3 | 8.5 | 3.316 | .001 |
| Nurses | 96 | 42.8 | 8.5 | 1.681 | .05 |
| Psychologists | 96 | 44.4 | 8.3 | .466 | .32 |
| Paraprofessionals | 95 | 44.9 | 9.3 | — | — |
| Social Workers | 140 | 45.5 | 9.4 | −.414 | .34 |

[*] Excludes 96 respondents in four minor occupational categories because of small N size.
[+] Highest possible activism score = 90; lowest possible activism score = 18.

An examination of personal/professional role, however, (Table 1) reveals some significant differences. Psychiatrists and nurses—both representative of medical education and socialization—are significantly less activist in their role conceptions than paraprofessionals. The paraprofessional appears to more closely approximate social workers and psychologists in this dimension.

A further examination of interprofessional differences (Table 2) reveals that paraprofessionals exceed all other workers in role discrepancy except social workers. In both Tables 1 and 2, however, these differences, although statistically significant, are quite small compared with both the actual range and potential range of the role measurement.

Table 2

Role Discrepancy Between
Paraprofessionals and Other Workers[*]

| Worker Affiliation | N | X[+] | SD | t test between paraprofessionals and each group of workers | P (One tail) |
|---|---|---|---|---|---|
| Psychiatrists ............... | 72 ........ | 3.14 ........ | 3.55 ........ | 5.33 ........ | .0001 |
| Psychologists ............... | 96 ........ | 5.45 ........ | 4.64 ........ | 2.15 .......... | .03 |
| Social Workers | 140 ........ | 6.49 ........ | 5.69 .......... | .69 .......... | .49 |
| Nurses ......................... | 96 ........ | 5.06 ........ | 3.99 ........ | 2.84 ........ | .005 |
| Paraprofessionals ...... | 95 ........ | 7.00 ........ | 5.32 ........... | — .......... | — |

[*] Excludes 96 respondents in four minor occupational categories because of small N size.
[+] Highest possible role discrepancy score = 72; lowest possible role discrepancy score = 0.

Up to this point, the authors have considered interoccupational differences in role perception and role discrepancy. It has also been indicated, however, the importance of understanding differences in the endorsement of community mental health ideology (CMHI). The CMHI was measured by use of the Baker-Schulberg Scale (1967) and comparison of professionals with paraprofessionals yields some interesting results. Basically, the professionals and paraprofessionals are similarly-grouped in the second and third quartiles of the CMHI. The professionals, however, exhibit a larger range of scores and a larger standard deviation. The professionals endorse CMHI at a significantly higher level than the paraprofessionals. This unexpected finding will be further discussed in the conclusions section.

Even though comparing professionals and paraprofessionals in CMHI revealed a statistically significant differ-

Table 3

CMHI Scores of Paraprofessionals and Other Workers[*]

| Affiliation | N | X[+] SD | t test between parapro- fessionals and each group of workers | P (one tail) |
|---|---|---|---|---|
| Psychiatrists .............. | 72 ...... 194.8 ........ 31.1 | ........ 2.83 | | ........ .002 |
| Paraprofessionals ...... | 95 ...... 207.4 ........ 26.2 | ............— | | ........— |
| Nurses ........................ | 96 ...... 210.2 ........ 28.8 | .. −0.689 | | ........ .214 |
| Psychologists .............. | 96 ...... 218.8 ........ 23.2 | .... −3.19 | | ........ .001 |
| Social Workers .......... | 140 ...... 220.9 ........ 26.4 | .... −3.85 | | ....... .0001 |

[*] Excludes 96 respondents in four minor occupational categories because of small N size.
[+] Highest possible score = 266; lowest possible score = 38.

ence, the necessity for more detailed comparison remains. This can be seen in Table 3. Interestingly, paraprofessionals are second only to psychiatrists in *low* endorsement of the CMHI. They endorse CMHI at a significantly lower level than psychologists and social workers. Their scores on the CMHI are not statistically different from nurses, the second least endorsing of the professional groups. Paraprofessionals, therefore, do not appear to constitute a source of ideological fervor or change in the CMHC.

None of the personal variables (age, sex, level of education) are significantly associated with CMHC paraprofessional activism. Sex and age, however, do make a difference in the personal/professional activism and role discrepancy of the paraprofessionals. Males are significantly higher in personal/professional activism and role discrepancy; those with a college degree or more education are higher in both measures than those with less education. This last finding is particularly noteworthy. *Those paraprofessionals, whose education makes them least like the indigenous populations from which they were presumably drawn, define the personal/professional role with greater activism.* In fact, their mean score exceeds the personal/professional mean activism for any professional group in the CMHC with the exception social workers.

The authors believed that the CMHC work experiences of paraprofessionals (time at CMHC and proportion of time spent in direct and indirect services) would be related to role activism and discrepancy. There is no evidence that paraprofessionals define the role differently, with regard to activism or have variation in role discrepancy as a function of time at the center. *This would indicate that their basic similarity to professionals is a characteristic with which they enter the center and not a product of co-optation.* The only work experience related to role definition seems to be the greater time spent on indirect services (community activities) is positively associated at a significant level with greater personal/-professional activism. Other research shows this also to be the case with other CMHC staff (Robin and Wagenfeld, 1976).

Earlier, the authors raised the question of whether the nature of the catchment area would affect the role definition and discrepancy of the paraprofessional. Although the paraprofessionals should be affected in two ways by the nature of the catchment areas—the social environment in which their center functions and the social environment from which they were recruited—no significant differences are seen. Urban, poverty, and catchment areas with greater proportions of black residents are not associated with paraprofessional activism or role discrepancy.[4]

---

[4] Analysis of data for paraprofessionals necessitated collapsing some of these organizational and catchment area characteristics.

With respect to organizational characteristics of the CMHC and paraprofessionals' role activism and discrepancy, the only significant association is between role discrepancy and center auspices. For the paraprofessional, the highest role discrepancy occurs in centers with public/governmental auspices; the lowest with agency/board auspices. It should be noted that public/governmental auspices; as the authors conceptualized it, included state mental hospitals, organizations that havetraditionally adopted a strong intramural approach to the provision of mental health services.[5] Agency/board auspices, on the other hand, have more often been the result of community coalitions for providing mental health services. As such, these auspices would probably be more receptive to manpower innovations.

In the prior analysis, the authors noted that variation in role definition and role discrepancy for paraprofessionals were associated with several sets of variables. Table 4 presents a stepwise multiple regression to specify which of the significant variables are associated with role definition and role discrepancy when they are viewed as a single predictive model. Since none of the variables predicted the paraprofessionals' CMHC activism, the analysis is confined to personal/professional activism and role discrepancy.

A total of 20% of the personal/professional activism was predicted by three significant variables; CMHI, education, and sex. CMHI is the strongest predictor ($R = .26$) followed by education and sex, each of which accounted for close to 3% of the variance. For the paraprofessional, therefore, there is the tendency for relatively abstract ideological commitment to be translated into role definition. Increased education and being male also adds to role activism.

In the role discrepancy of the paraprofessionals 22% of

---

[5] These organizations are also likely to define paraprofessional roles in a very restrictive or traditional manner.

Table 4

Stepwise Multiple Regression for CMHC Paraprofessionals: Personal/Professional Activism and Role Discrepancy by Predictor Variables

| | | Personal/Professional Activism | | |
| | | | Significance | |
| Added Variable | R | Increment F | P | Coefficient |
| --- | --- | --- | --- | --- |
| CMHI* | .26 | - ..... 6.73 | .01 | .09 |
| Education | .36 | .10 ..... 6.94 | .01 | -1.16 |
| Sex | .45 | .09 ..... 8.20 | .005 | -5.00 |

R = .45
R² = .20
F = 7.80
P = .0001

| | | | | Significance | |
| Added Variable | R | Increment F | P | Coefficient |
| --- | --- | --- | --- | --- |
| Education | .28 | - ..... 7.79 | .006 | -.72 |
| Sex | .38 | .10 ..... 7.52 | .007 | -2.8 |
| Geographic Complexity | .43 | .05 ..... 3.82 | .05 | -.80 |
| Auspices | .46 | .03 ..... 3.87 | .05 | -8.0 |

R = .46
R² = .22
F = 4.91
P = .0005

the variance was explained by four factors: education, sex, geographic complexity, and CMHC auspices.

Ideology plays no part in role discrepancy even though it is the strongest factor in predicting personal/professional activism. Education and sex, on the other hand, predict both in the same direction. It should be noted, parenthetically, that the level of prediction for the professionals (in data not presented here) is lower, and CMHC activism is predictable by substantially different variables than those of the paraprofessionals. Hence, it appears the professionals and paraprofessionals reach the same levels of activism and discrepancy by different routes.

## Conclusions

The data indicate that paraprofessionals do not define organizational role in a manner different from other staff at the CMHC. They differ significantly by defining their personal role with more activism than the medically trained staff, but not the rest of the CMHC staff. It seems more realistic to state that nurses and psychiatrists are notable for *their* differences from the rest of the staff— *including paraprofessionals*. The paraprofessionals exhibited more role discrepancy than all other major professional categories, with the exception of social workers. The putatively unique status of the paraprofessionals, however, does not yield the great role discrepancy that one might expect from persons brought into CMHC as community activists.

The comparisons of paraprofessionals to professionals indicate that the paraprofessionals do not bring activism into the CMHC at either a high absolute level or a level beyond that purveyed by most of the professionals. In abstract ideology, which presages role definition, the paraprofessionals are less inclined to support community mental health ideology than all the other professionals, with the exception of the medical staff. Have they been co-opted? The data yield no evidence of co-optation. Neither CMHC nor personal/professional activism decrease with time at the CMHC. Additionally, personal/professional activism *increases* with greater education. Were the paraprofessionals being co-opted through formal or center-connected educational opportunities, activism would decrease or—given its initial low level—remain the same. It appears that paraprofessionals, however, are being educated to the professionals' concept of activism from an initial low level of activism. This is supported by the significantly higher endorsement of CMHI by the more educated paraprofessionals.

Miller et al. (1970), assert that paraprofessionals are "creamed" by the CMHCs in order to select those persons with characteristics most similar to the professional staff. The relatively large proportion of paraprofessionals with bachelors degrees would seem to be supportive of this. In addition, the fact that they appear—in our measures of role—to be so similar to the professionals, lends additional credence.

Those advocating the use of paraprofessionals in CMHCs or other human service agencies argued that they could serve the important function of a bridge between the agency and the community. It is clear that if the paraprofessionals are co-opted (made different from the indigenous population from which they are drawn) or "creamed" (selected for their differences from the population from which they are drawn), their ability to serve as bridgemen is compromised. The data here show no evidence of co-optation, but supports the conclusion of creaming and, to that extent, call to task the paraprofessional in the CMHC as bridgeman.[6]

---

[6]These conclusions are predicted on the same assumption that serves as the major rationale for the creation of the paraprofessional: i.e., that the values and ideology of those *served* by the CMHCs are different from those professionals *providing* the service. The extent to which the professionals and paraprofessionals view the community as a locus of control is an indirect indicator of this. Data not presented in this article indicate that the paraprofessionals and professionals view the community differently in this regard.

What policy implications can be drawn from these data? Paraprofessionals were originally envisaged as serving a multiplicity of functions. They cannot, however, be all things to all centers. If they were hired to bring an element of activism into the CMHCs, the data do not support this intention. If the purpose was establishment of bridges with the indigenous population, the authors can question whether the more educated paraprofessionals (similar in role definition to the nonmedical professionals) are representative of their communities in the sense intended by architects of these programs. These data, confined to staff of CMHCs, do not allow the authors to describe the beliefs and role expectations of the CMHC's catchment area residents, so no closure can be effected on this point. The paraprofessional can, and still could, be quite viable as a bridgeperson in the CMHC by acting as liaison or interpreter between the client and professional therapist. Here, though, one could question the interpretive abilities of the more educated and professional-like paraprofessionals in performing this task.

In an editorial finale, Jackson (1975) made the comment that none of the manuscripts crossing her desk regarding paraprofessionals in human services programs continued to romanticize this group. It seems clear that the Rousseauean aura applied to the paraprofessional by those supporting their cause has been considerably muted. (Also see: Franklin Arnhoff's "New Careers: Where Have All the Flowers Gone?" in this volume.) The first flush of enthusiasm has given way to disenchantment on both sides. As Ritzer (1974) has noted, paraprofessionals are beginning to organize, unionize, and otherwise follow the paths traditionally made by other developing occupational groups. Paraprofessionals have also expressed their dissatisfaction through strikes and "revolts" (e.g., Health/PAC, 1971), but the sources of discontent might have been self-, rather than, collectively-oriented.

It would be erroneous to regard this article as a rejection of the *concept* of paraprofessionals in CMHCs. Rather, it would be more appropriate to say that data here suggest manifest activist and community bridging purposes intended by theoreticians and program planners, do not seem to have been realized. Future programs predicated on these beliefs and expectations, then, should be viewed with some skepticism. This lack of *activism*, however, could also be viewed in a positive light as a possible index of integration with the professional staff. The paraprofessional does not appear to be a source of great organizational strain.

Advocates of paraprofessionals (e.g., Pearl and Riessman, 1965; Reiff, 1964) have argued that they can be an important pool of manpower, and that jobs for them in human services programs can represent a meaningful way out of poverty. This view of the paraprofessional seems supported. They are similar to the professional and, hence, not "upsetting." They are relatively inexpensive and, for some segment of the indigenous population, employment is provided.

For other social activist purposes, however, paraprofessionals will have to be selected specifically. The category itself insures no more activism than most of the professional categories. When activist or bridgeman paraprofessionals are selected, then the center administrators can begin to worry about disruption or co-optation; at this point, the concern seems premature and superfluous.

REFERENCE NOTES

1.  The data presented here is part of a larger study "Emerging Roles of Community Mental Health Workers," supported by grant MH18958, from the National Institute of Mental Health.

REFERENCES

Ahearn, F. L. Paraprofessionals: Anomie and activism. Paper presented at the National Conference of Social Welfare, Chicago, 1970.

Albee, G.W. *Mental health manpower trends*. New York: Basic Books, 1959.

Albrecht, G.L. The indigenous mental health worker: The cure-all for what ailment. In Roman & Trice (Eds.), *The Sociology of Psychotherapy*. New York: Jason Aronson, 1974.

Arnhoff, F., Jenkins, J., & Speisman, J. The new mental health workers. In F. Arnhoff, E. Rubenstein, & J. Speisman (Eds.), *Manpower for mental health*. Chicago: Aldine Publishing Co., 1969b.

Baker, F., & Schulberg, H. The development of a community mental health ideology scale. *Community Mental Health Journal*, 1967, 3, 216-225.

Boyette, R., Blount, W., & Petaway, K. The plight of the new careerist. *American Journal of Orthopsychiatry*, 1971, 49 *XLI*, 237-238.

Christmas, J.J. Group methods in training and practice: Nonprofessional mental health personnel in a deprived community. *American Journal of Orthopsychiatry*, 1966, *35*, 410-419

David, H. A perspective on manpower theory and conceptualization. In F. Arnhoff, E. Rubenstein, & J. Speisman (Eds.), *Manpower for Mental Health*. Chicago: Aldine Publishing Co., 1969.

Geiger, C. Ideology as a cultural system. In *Ideology and dissent*, New York: Free Press, 1967.

Haug, M. R. & Sussman, M. B. Professional autonomy and the revolt of the client. *Social Problems*, 1969, *17*, 153-161.

Health-Pac *The American health empire: Power, profits, and politics*. New York: Vintage Books, 1971.

Jackson, J.J. Some special concerns about race and health: An editorial finale. *Journal of Health and Social Behavior*, 1975, *16*, 342-428.

Joint Commission on Mental Illness and Health. *Final Report: Action for mental health*. New York: Science Editions, 1961.

Littlestone, R. Mental health manpower planning. In R.

278 PARAPROFESSIONALS IN THE HUMAN SERVICES

McKnickle & M. Higman (Eds.), *Regional Mental Health Planning Conference*, Portland, Ore., 1964.

McKnickle, R., & Higman, M. *Regional Mental Health Planning Conference*, Portland, Ore., 1964.

Miller, S.M., Robey, P. and Steenwijk, A. Creaming the poor. *Transaction*, 1970, *7* (June), 38-45.

Minuchin, S. The paraprofessional and the use of confrontation in the mental health field. *American Journal of Orthopsychiatry*, 1969, *39*, 722-729.

Pearl, A. and Riessman, R. (Eds.), *New careers for the poor*. New York: Free Press, 1965.

Riessman, F. The revolution in social work: The new nonprofessional. New York. *Mobilization for Youth Report*, 1963.

Riley, W. The paraprofessional polemic: Investigating the case of the paraprofessional in the community mental health center. M.A. thesis, Western Michigan University, 1976.

Ritzer, G. Indigenous nonprofessionals in community mental health: Boon or boondoggle. In P. Roman & H. Trice, *The Sociology of Psychotherapy*. New York: Jason Aronson, 1974.

Robin, S. & Wagenfeld, M. The nature and correlates of community mental health ideology in community mental health centers. *Journal of Community Psychology*, 1976, *4*, 335-340.

Robin, S. & Wagenfeld, M. The community mental health worker: Organizational and personal sources of role discrepancy. *Journal of Health and Social Behavior*, 1977, *18*, 16-26.

Torrey, E. F. The case of the indigenous therapist. *Archives of General Psychiatry*, 1969, *20*, 365-373.

Wagenfeld, M., Robin, S. & Jones, J. Structural and professional correlates of ideologies of community mental health workers. *Journal of Health and Social Behavior*, 1974, *15*, (3), 199-210.

Willcox, P. The new professionals: Practical aspects of the use of new careerists in public health agencies. *Mental Hygiene*, 1970, *20*, 373-396.

# Paraprofessionals in the Home

Allana Cumming Elovson, Ph. D.
*Home Start, San Diego, California*

## INTRODUCTION

Ann O'Keefe, Ed.D.
*National Home Start Director*
*(1971-1978)*

*Home Start is a form of Head Start. Staff in Head Start centers, on one hand, provide a comprehensive child development program designed to offer children a wide and rich array of opportunities, activities, and services (including health services and social services for the child's family).*

*Staff of a Home Start program, on the other hand, work directly with parents to help them do, or provide, for their own children, at home, the same kinds of activities, experiences and services that are provided to children who attend Head Start centers. Thus, the Home Start concept builds on the recognition that parents—for better or for worse—are, in fact, the first and most important influences on a child's life. This increased awareness on the part of parents often helps them to be even more helpful and supportive to their children as they grow and develop.*

*Although Home Start usually eschews the term "paraprofessional" to describe its largely non college graduate home visitors, the fact is that often, the Home Visitor represents the pinnacle of paraprofessionalism. Thus, after stating as one of its conclusions that the Home Start demonstration showed that "Paraprofessionals can be effective providers of Home Start services," the Home Start Evaluation report went on to say, "They (Home Visitors) played a key role . . . and did the work of professionals. In fact, not being professional was viewed by many project staff as an asset, making it easier to establish a close and trusting relationship with parents." (Love, et al., 1976).*

*The author of this chapter, Dr. Elovson, has been the director of the Home Start program in San Diego since its beginning in 1973 as one of the 16 demonstration programs funded by HEW.*

## THE BEGINNING OF HOME START

From March, 1972 to June, 1975 the Administration for Children, Families and, Youth conducted a nationwide demonstration program called Home Start. At each of the 16 different locations comprising the overall program, paraprofessionals, through the medium of home visits, brought comprehensive child development and family support services directly to the homes of low income families, from diverse backgrounds who had young children. While all of the 16 programs pursued common goals, they were selected in a variety of locations and differed from each other in many fundamental ways. In all of these programs, however, paraprofessionals working in the home have been the backbone of the operation. In effect, the Home Start demonstration has served as a proving ground where much has been learned about the use of paraprofessionals in home-based programs.

In order to understand how paraprofessionals have been used in the Home Start program and continue to be used in similar home-based activities throughout the country, as well as to examine the extent to which what has been learned from these programs can be put to good use in others, it is necessary to first understand something about how and why the Home Start program was begun and implemented. Moreover, it is essential to examine what is known of its achievements and problems at this time. The following is an account of the origins of Home Start, the way in which it has realized its goals, how paraprofessionals have functioned in the program, how effective they have been, and what has been found necessary to establish and support their effectiveness in these and similar programs.

In 1971, the Office of Child Development, under the leadership of its first director Dr. Edward Zigler, decided to launch a new kind of Head Start program. The program would be both home-based and parent-focused, and would be designed to help parents do with their own children at home the same kinds of things that Head Start staff do with children in Head Start centers. While Head Start had, from its very beginning, given a great deal of emphasis to "parent involvement" as one component of its child development program,[1] this new Home Start program sought to involve parents as the *major* means of

[1] In addition to parent involvement the other program components of Head Start are Education (Child Development); Health; which includes physical, dental and mental health, Nutrition Safety; and Social Services.

providing children with their own Head Start in their own home.

The decision to create a parent-focused program was also shaped by several factors. In many of the precursor home-based programs which preceded the national Home Start demonstration it was most often the case that the traveling teacher or nurse worked directly with the child. It was not unusual for the child's mother to retire to another area of the home while the visiting "teacher" tutored the child. There was, however, a growing body of evidence (Gray and Klaus, 1970; Gordon, 1971; Klaus and Gray, 1968; Levenstein, 1970; Shaefer, 1968; and Weikart, et al., 1970) suggesting that the most effective programs were those in which the staff focused not on the child, but rather on the parents, who could then, themselves, carry out needed activities with the child after the visitor left. There was also increasing recognition within Head Start that there needed to be ongoing support and reinforcement at home, by parents, for what children were doing and learning at the center, as well as a desire for increased parental involvement directly in children's development.

By March, 1972, Dr. Ann O'Keefe was appointed National Director of Home Start, sites had been selected, and 15 Home Start programs established throughout the country.[2] All were adjuncts of existing Head Start programs or community action agencies. The purpose of these programs was to build on existing family strengths by assisting parents in their roles as their children's first, and most important, teachers. They were to bring to enrolled families the same range of services provided by the Head Start program, but in addition, they were to build parent's confidence and abilities to provide their own children with the same developmental experiences provided at Head Start centers. In fact, due to the unique nature of the program, and the particular synergism of

[2]San Diego, the 16th Program, was not begun until January 1973.

its combined parent-focused and home-based features, many of the programs went quite beyond those aims and created a new and special type of program: Home Start.

The Home Start Guidelines, specified that the program objectives were to 1) involve parents directly in the education of their children, 2) help strengthen parents' capacity for facilitating their children's development, 3) demonstrate methods of delivering comprehensive Head Start services to children and parents (or surrogate parents) for whom a center-based program was not feasible, and 4) compare the relative costs and benefits of center and home-based comprehensive early child development programs in areas where both types of programs were feasible.

Although the goals of all these programs were similar, the problems to be solved in reaching them were different. Consequently, the roles played by the paraprofessional staff were diverse. In all cases, and in all settings, it was paraprofessionals who made visits and it was the paraprofessionals who became the Home Start program. In large measure, it has been the paraprofessionals on whom the programs' achievement has depended.

## The Decision to use Paraprofessionals

Although the original guidelines did not explicitly specify the use of paraprofessionals as home visitors, (they did direct, however, that where feasible, trained Head Start parents should be used) there were a number of factors which made it necessary, inevitable and, ultimately, highly desirable to do so. Before these reasons are presented, however, a functional definition of a paraprofessional should be considered. Paraprofessionals are usually considered to be persons without college degrees and/or the advanced training in a particular field of study that enables them to function at a professional level. It has, however, proved considerably more serviceable, at least in the San Diego Home Start program, to regard a paraprofessional as someone for whom the the specific set of abilities and skills needed by a home visitor cannot be assumed on the basis of specialized training. By such a definition, persons with college degrees, and even those with more advanced training in certain areas, (such as chemistry, mathematics, or business administration) could be regarded, and expected to function, even after training, as paraprofessionals in jobs such as parent counselor, home aide, or home visitor. This, in fact, has proven to be true and clearly has many implications for the selection and training of paraprofessionals.

A number of considerations led to the decision to use paraprofessionals as home visitors (or family advocates as they are often called). Perhaps the first among these was that there simply was no such thing as a *professional* home visitor. Although the jobs of home visitors resembled each other in some respects from locale to locale, there really had not been, prior to the Home Start demonstration, a clearly defined job such as home visitor, nor were there at that time any systematic training programs, at any level, specifically for such a job, professional or otherwise. This meant that there were no pool of professional Home Visitors upon which to draw.

Certainly, there were many professionals in the fields allied to the Home Visitor's function, such as preschool teachers, child psychologists, and social workers who could have been able to meet the requirements of the role of home visitor as it evolved. For a number of reasons, however, it was not very likely that many of these professionals would be found who would be willing to assume the role. For one thing, the budgets allotted to each program precluded payment of salaries anywhere within a professional range.

Another factor that ruled out the use of professionals as home visitors concerned the nature of the job itself. The job of the home visitor was too varied and many-sided to fit the kind of training most professionals had had. Essentially, the job consists of helping families acquire whatever services, information, and materials are necessary for them to meet their needs, almost whatever these may be. It requires visitors to be able to bring information and help families acquire services in a number of different areas (health, nutrition, childhood education, and community resources): it does *not* require them to provide in-depth services at a professional level in any one of these areas, as would be emphasized by the training most professionals receive. The job of home visitor often requires driving ten to twenty hours a week to make visits, to walk through hot and dusty (and sometimes icy) country roads; to climb tenement stairs, to demonstrate toothbrushing and to help change a baby, to wait in welfare offices, immunization clinics, emergency and court rooms, and to circle supermarket aisles pushing a cart to read labels and demonstrate comparison shopping. It would have been very difficult to find conventionally-trained professionals for such jobs at modest salaries.

There were a number of other factors, relating to the populations being served that suggested the *desirability* of using paraprofessionals. The families in the Home Start program had to meet the same income eligibility requirements as those who were enrolled in Head Start. This meant that families had incomes at, or below, federal poverty guidelines. A large proportion of these families (35%) were non white and drawn from a variety of different ethnic, cultural, and language backgrounds. Many of them spoke no English, received no services of this kind before, and had had extremely limited contact with the majority culture. It seemed likely that families would relate best to persons whom they felt understood their points of view, spoke their language, knew local ways, and had had many of the same experiences.

Other factors fundamental to program goals pointed clearly to the use of paraprofessionals as not only desirable but *crucial* to the Home Start program. Since participation in the program was purely voluntary on the part of the families, and since the goal of the Home Visitor was to help parents, week by week, step by step, to develop the skills and self-confidence to become effective agents of change in their own lives, it was clear that the visitor would have to *take* and *maintain*, over the long haul, a low-power position, quite subordinate to the position of parents in their own home. Establishing such a relationship of equality or subordination might well have proven difficult, if at all possible, using professionals, since families might view them with too much awe and feel intimidated by them. Moreover, a central feature of the job of home visitor is that of the model. In every visit the home visitor models in countless ways: she/he models how to use and make educational toys, or what may very well be totally new ways of interacting positively with children. She models how to plan a budget, how to be effective and assertive in dealing with authorities, and how to take one's life in one's own hands. As research has shown (Bandura and Walters, 1963) for models to be effective in bringing about behavioral changes, it must be possible for observers to identify somehow with that model, to see that someone, like themselves, can do certain things. Clearly, professionals assuring families that family members can do the same things as the professional simply cannot have the same kind of persuasive effect as can someone whom the families see as very much like themselves doing it, and doing it successfully, right in front of their eyes.

Taken together, these considerations lead inexorably to the decision to use paraprofessionals in the Home Start program, a decision that has served the program well.

## How Paraprofessionals Have Functioned in the Home Start Program as Home Visitors

As is evident by the above, paraprofessionals have been central to the Home Start program. Despite the differences among programs, they have been the principal means of bringing a wide range of individualized services to families. To many families, paraprofessionals as home visitors *are* the Home Start program, and in many ways and on many levels this has been true.

Home visitors have performed so many different kinds of tasks that it would perhaps be most useful to recount these in terms of the *types* of different things they have done as well as in terms of the different *kinds* of roles they have played. Before doing so, however, it is necessary to preface this by stating that these functions are those that have been performed by *trained* home visitors. It must be stressed that adequate training, both pre-service and continuing inservice, is essential for adequate performance of these roles.

Basically, the job of the paraprofessional visitor in Home Start has included recruiting families, determining their eligibility and enrolling them, explaining the scope of the program, assessing children's needs and those of the individual family members, and helping meet those needs. Each visitor typically carried a caseload of from between 10 and 15 families[3] whose visits were planned and recorded each week. The Home Start Evaluation showed that visits lasted approximately 1½ hours and incorporated activities from several components, as described above.

In the San Diego Home Start Program, program personnel have identified more than 12 different roles which home visitors play from time to time (sometimes several in the same day). No doubt, a similar analysis of home visitors' activities in similar programs would yield others as well.

The first of these, directly concerned with the home visits themselves, involves that of being an *information*

[3] Home Start Final Evaluation Findings indicate that Home Visitors working with more than 13 families had difficulty maintaining frequent and regular contact with families resulting in a decline in child development in the areas of school readiness and language development.

*provider.* On a typical visit, the home visitor brings information and/or materials relating to the family's needs in several component areas. They also demonstrate how to *use* these materials, discuss what these pamphlets mean, and relate the information to the specific children in the home and the specific problems parents have. They make parents aware of the range of resources available in the community that can help them meet their needs—from immunization to recreation or job counseling. They show parents how to make toys and other educational materials from things around their homes, and how everyday household activities can be used as important educational experiences for their children. During the course of a visit, the home visitor will also function as a *model* for the parents, usually in her manner of interacting with children and in her way of using the materials she has brought.

Since home visits present unparalleled opportunities for observation of both the families' day-to-day functioning, their resources, and their interpersonal interaction patterns, the home visitor also functions as an *observer* and *information gatherer* of the kind of data that can never be obtained by office interviews or standardized testing. Moreover, the opportunity for ongoing weekly observation of children in their own homes, has made home visitors successful in identifying incipient conditions needing special attention, such as handicaps unrecognized up to that time.

Still another function expertly performed by home visitors has been that of *outreach worker* in the community. This role has emerged as a result of home visitors' functioning as a link between the parents and community agencies. Moreover, it has enabled parents to learn about and obtain services they need. Paraprofessionals have been found to function extremely effectively as *facilitators* for parents once they have decided to use the services of various agencies. Often, paraprofessionals accompany families to agencies. There, they interpret, attend interviews, assist families in filling out forms and, in general, help the parents shape the experiences into positive ones. In many situations, home visitors function actively as *advocates* for families. They help untangle the delays, mixups, and errors which sometimes occur in obtaining services.

Conversely, home visitors also function as *sources of information* or *resources* to many agencies in the community regarding the family in ways that have sometimes been quite crucial for some families. With the families' consent, and following consultations with Home Start supervisory personnel, home visitors have often attended case conferences, staff meetings at hospitals and clinics, and court hearings. Here, they contribute their particular information and insights relating to the families. These insights are especially valuable as they are available only to those who have had the opportunities for observation provided by the special relationship of the home visitor to the family. This includes their repeated observations of the family in their own home.

Another role that paraprofessionals have performed very successfully in Home Start has been as a *channel between professionals* or special consultants *to the family.* They assist families to implement the instructions or directions given by specialists, and show them how to carry them out at home. This has proven especially useful in situations where there is a handicapping condition that requires the parents to provide special kinds of therapeutic experiences at home or to follow a particular regime. On returning home from the specialist's office, the home visitor has often assisted parents to see how these activities could actually be carried out at home. They help parents decide just where to attach the pulley, which table could be used for exercises, and just *how* to smear peanut butter on a child's lip as the speech therapist directed. The author has found home visitors to be extremely effective in helping families identify and use resources in themselves and in their own homes.

Home visitors, of course, frequently *transport* families to and from badly needed services they could not otherwise obtain. Typically, they use the transportation and waiting time to discuss many of the same things they would at a visit. As Home Start programs began to provide activities for families other than in their own homes, the home visitors often took on the role of *organizers* and group facilitators of special meetings, such as play groups, field trips, and special classes for parents and children. In the San Diego Home Start program, home visitors sometimes work together in pairs to arrange special events for families on a particular topic or at a particular location. They survey parents' needs and interests, arrange for speakers on particular topics, and obtain nearby places in the community where these activities can be held. In addition, home visitors often pool their individual skills and draw upon them directly. One home visitor, with experience as a Berlitz instructor, held classes to teach parents the English essential for them to obtain and hold jobs, as the services had not been available in the community when and where they had been needed.

In the San Diego Home Start program, the author has found that home visitors can also materially assist with research and evaluation. In this program, the pretesting and assessment activities are meshed, and as soon as home visitors have established effective relationships with their families, they administer the pretest survey instruments the author and her associates designed to assess the families' entering level of information in the various component areas. These data are then used to develop a plan for home visits as well as to provide a baseline to judge later progress.

Paraprofessionals in Home Start have also functioned as *representatives of the program* to other agencies, many times attending special meetings held with other agency staff to inform them about the range of services Home

Start provides. Often, they visit meetings of local charitable organizations to enlist support and donations.

Finally, when it comes time for children to make the transition to the public school, the author has found that the home visitor can function very effectively as a *bridge between the family and the public school.* They arrange and attend a meeting that includes the parents, child, teacher, and principal. Here, all parties can first make each others' acquaintance in a relaxed atmosphere, as equal partners in the child's future development.

This description of some of the many different roles and functions of home visitors in the San Diego Home Start program has been used to demonstrate the variety, flexibility, and skill with which carefully selected, well-trained paraprofessionals can effectively function in programs such as these.[4]

## THE EFFECTIVENESS OF HOME START

Considering all the things done by the paraprofessional in Home Start, one's most immediate response might be to ask: How effective is this program, literally built on use of paraprofessionals in the home?

Since one of the major program objectives specified in the original Home Start guidelines was to determine the relative costs and benefits of center and home-based comprehensive child development programs, the Home Start demonstration program has been extensively evaluated. The results of this evaluation have been extremely useful in illuminating the ways in which the program has been effective and some crucial factors in its effectiveness.

At the initiation of the Home Start Demonstration, contracts were issued to the High-Scope Educational Re-

[4]The reader who wishes to know how paraprofessionals have been used in other Home Start programs can find such information in the extensive material produced by the formative evaluation, all of which is available through ERIC.

search Foundation and Abt Associates to conduct a major evaluation to run parallel with the demonstration program. The research design, developed by Esther Kresh, Administration for Children, Youth and Family's Home Start Evaluation Officer, focused on the effects of Home Start on both children and parents.

The design of the Home Start evaluation incorporated three distinct components: 1) an information system; 2) a formative, or process, evaluation in which all of the 16 Home Start programs participated; and 3) a summative or impact evaluation, which was conducted at six sites. The summative evaluation was designed to provide information about Home Start's overall effectiveness by measuring a variety of changes in parents and children compared to both a randomly selected, delayed-entry control group, and comparable groups of children within center based Head Start programs.

Pre and post measurements were collected at the six summative sites each October and May, beginning in May, 1973. Thus, such data were obtained four times during the course of the demonstration, following periods of 7, 12, and 20 months after the pre-test in the fall of 1973. The final phase of the evaluation (1974-75) included a comparison of program impact after one and two years of program involvement as well as the replication of the seventh month findings.[5]

In general, Home Start evaluation findings provided convincing evidence of the effectiveness of a parent-focused home-based child development program using paraprofessionals. Although these results do not speak specifically to the use of paraprofessionals compared to professionals in home-based programs, (that was not a focus of the research design) the data do indicate differ-

---

[5] All reports prepared by the evaluation contractors during this 3½ years of Home Start are available through the ERIC system. A listing of these reports, and their ERIC identification numbers, can be found in the Home Start Evaluation Final Report, 1976, available from Home Start Administration for Children, Youth and Family.

ences in impact between programs using paraprofessionals in center-based and home-based programs. They show that using paraprofessionals in the home is at least as effective as using them in center settings. Although complete discussion of the data of the home-based programs compared to both the Head Start population and to the control groups is not possible here, certain aspects of these findings are of particular relevance to the use of paraprofessionals in home-based programs. The results for Home Start children were, on a number of measures, significantly better than those of the control group and were generally comparable to the results for Head Start center-based children.[6] In both comparisons, however, there were significant differences in certain aspects of the parental behavior assessed. The 7-month findings showed that Home Start mothers were more likely than control group mothers to encourage their children to help with household tasks, taught more pre-reading and pre-writing skills to their children, provided more books and playthings, and had more positive interactions with them during the course of the day than did control group parents. Home Start mothers were more likely to employ a teaching style involving thought-provoking questions, to engage in a higher rate of verbal interaction in that situation, and to focus their talk around dimensions of the tasks. In addition, at both the 7 and 12 month intervals, Home Start children continued to show significant differences from control group children on the Caldwell Pre-

---

[6] At the end of the first 7-month period, the major differences between the Head Start and Home Start groups were in the areas of *nutrition, immunizations, day care*, and *"things mothers teach their children"*. With regard to the first three, Head Start children fared significantly better on the nutrition food intake measure (due in large part to the fact that center-based children were receiving food on a daily basis), had more immunizations (100% of the center-based children had been fully immunized), and received day care services (which were not usually necessary for Home Start families). *However, Home Start mothers did more "teaching" to their own children than did Head Start mothers.*

school Inventory, a nationally used school-readiness measure.

The thoroughness and the complexity of the 3½ year evaluation of Home Start permits no easy generalizations or simple conclusions regarding Home Start in comparison to the two other groups. It can be said, however, that the Home Start program, using paraprofessionals to deliver a wide variety of comprehensive child development and family support services, has been demonstrated as being especially effective in influencing styles of parent child interaction in the direction of increased parent functioning as "teachers" to their children.

The most important aspect of the findings is that the Home Start program has been particularly effective in accomplishing the special goals of the program; to assist parents to become more active and effective teachers of their own children in their own homes and it has been through the use of paraprofessionals in the home that this goal has been realized.

## CHARACTERISTICS OF HOME VISITORS

Much has been learned about the home visitors who made these results possible and about the kind of characteristics that define the "ideal" visitor. The paraprofessionals who have worked as home visitors in Home Start have been almost exclusively female (only three males worked in Home Start as home visitors, and only one as long as a year). They range in age from 18 to 59, with an average age of 34. This predominance of women has been due in large part to a strong cultural resistance to men working alone with married women in their homes. There is also a scarcity of men working on the direct service level in child development programs largely due to the extremely low salaries paid for such jobs as well as to role expectations. During the period of the Home Start demonstration (1972-1975), 32% of these visitors were drawn from non-white populations reflecting, as closely as possible, the ethnic composition of the families whom they served. In most cases, the average home visitor had been previously employed in a job which was in some way related to her job in the Home Start program.

Only half the visitors in Home Start had any formal education beyond high school and only 10% had college degrees. Of this 10% only a small percentage had any prior background in child development. In terms of general effectiveness, however, the author believes it is important to stress that although research data report no measurable difference in the effectiveness of home visitors who had college degrees and those who did not, it has been my personal experience that home visitors with some college background in child development were more effective than those who came without this background. Although there has been apprehension that home visitors with "too much education" would be unable to relate well to families due to social class differences in values and perspective, this has not been the author's experience. Moreover it has not been always necessary to have home visitors of the same racial and ethnic background as the families they serve. When the San Diego Home Start began, guidelines directed the recruitment of white, black, Mexican-American, Japanese, Chinese, Filipino, and Samoan-Guamanian families, as well as Navy families with parents of different racial and ethnic backgrounds. Accordingly, a white, black, Mexican-American, Chinese, Japanese, and Filipino home visitor were hired. (We were unable to obtain any Samoan or Guamanian visitors.) When it was necessary to serve across these categories, home visitors experienced no rejection on racial grounds. The Japanese visitor was easily accepted by both Samoan and Filipino families. At other times, both the Filipino and Chinese visitors were fully accepted by both white and black families.

A certain set of factors seem to characterize those paraprofessionals who become effective home visitors. Among these are good mental and physical health, energy and patience, optimism, common sense, resourcefulness, humor, and a strong motivation to work with people. The ideal home visitor is one who understands, either through her own experience, or through training, imagination and/or empathy, both the difficult circumstances in which many Home Start families live and the inevitable impact of these circumstances on the families' attitudes, behavior, and aspirations. Although the home visitor may not necessarily have suffered the same kind of poverty or feelings of social alienation, she is able to understand the deprivation of the families with whom she works. She sees them in terms of a complex set of circumstances rather than as people with personal, moral, or intellectual failings. Basic to her effectiveness is a nonjudgmental and supportive attitude. She is aware of how families such as those enrolled in Home Start, stand outside the usual channels for obtaining information relevant to their needs. The ideal visitor has been found to be a person who is an extremely good listener and can avoid directly giving advice, while presenting alternatives and information.

No matter how much background she already brings to the job, an effective home visitor is one who clearly demonstrates an interest and ability to learn and an awareness that there *are* things to learn. A sensitivity to cultural values and styles of personal interaction, whether brought to the job or acquired as part of her training, has also been found to be essential. A communication style that is constructive and empathetic rather than critical and directive, and a warm, friendly but not over-powering style are important. The most effective home visitors are those who, though friendly and deeply concerned with assisting families to learn to solve their problems, can maintain the kind of objective, professional attitude necessary to help, from the outside, rather than becoming too involved to be useful.

It has been found that effective home visitors are those

who have other sources of satisfaction in their lives. They do not depend upon the responsiveness of families, their gratitude, and their changes in the "right direction" for their own self esteem. Consequently, effective home visitors are those who are *constantly* alert to avoid creating dependency in the families with whom they work. They strive to build families' ability to help themselves. Characteristic of the ideal home visitor in Home Start is an ability to respond flexibly to situations and opportunities as they arise, and to use them in the interests of the family. The successful home visitor has been one who is not afraid of working with the staffs of other community agencies and is able to build the kind of relationship with their staffs which permits her to be an effective advocate for the families with whom she works.

In addition to this list of impressive, but highly necessary, personal qualities, an effective home visitor must also be able to complete what is often a great amount of necessary paper work, organize time efficiently, work most of the week without close supervision and keep a careful record of her activities in order to determine whether or not she and the family are achieving their objectives. When one adds to this the indispensable qualities of abundant good sense, perseverance, resourcefulness, maturity, optimism, and a sense of humor, it is clear that personal qualities figure perhaps more importantly as training, credentials, and experience in the ideal visitor. This makes the *selection* of visitors a critical aspect of the program.

Due to the nature of home visiting, the most important single factor in its success is the paraprofessionals who do the home visiting. Since it is not possible to overstress the importance of the home visitors, themselves, their selection should receive the utmost attention and involve the greatest skill and judgment possible. Few aspects of the program will so amply repay the care and effort exerted, in few other aspects of the program will poor decisions so drastically penalize program operations. Since many of the characteristics crucial to the ideal home visitor are personal ones, no amount of subsequent training, supervision, or on-the-job experience can fully compensate for improper selection.

Since the particular factors that make a good home visitor, such as commitment, empathy, conscientiousness, patience and respect for the families with whom they work, cannot be predicted from factors such as education or even previous experience, they are extremely difficult to gauge from the information required by most job application forms. Finding paraprofessionals with the characteristics necessary for home visitors requires considerably more interviewing than is necessary for jobs whose performance can more easily be predicted from prior training. Consequently, job applications and personal statements of qualifications should be carefully scrutinized for indications of activities suggesting strong interest or commitment to this kind of work and for some valuable skills. It would be foolish to believe, however, even after five years of Home Start experience, that a systematic, objective and reliable method to select home visitors has been developed. In the San Diego program, the procedure typically involves three interviews. The first is with the supervisory staff who screen applications. The second is usually with the home visiting and other support staff, and the third with families currently enrolled in the program.

During the interview, the applicants were evaluated by their 1) attitude toward the poor; 2) concept of the role of home visitor; 3) awareness that the job involves primarily working with parents and to a lesser extent with children; 4) experience, at any level, with young children and her awareness of some of the difficulties of being a parent; 5) ability and willingness to learn, and the recognition that at least some training would be necessary before beginning home visiting; 6) ability to recognize that change takes time, and the ability to persevere even when nothing much appears to be happening; 7) lack of need for others' dependence and gratitude; 8) adequate basic skills of reading, mathematics and writing; 9) recognition of the importance of careful record keeping; of filling out forms, daily logs, etc.; 10) non-obtrusive self-presentation; 11) good health, and willingness to work very hard; and 12) recognition of the central importance of parents to children's lives. Because of space limitations, it is not possible here to discuss these 12 factors found to be useful in the selection of home visitors. They are included here as an indication of the kinds of things that an interview for selecting paraprofessionals for home visiting programs might seek to assess.

At this point, the reader might well be wondering if setting such high standards and taking so many pains in the selection process is realistic. The question arises, too, of whether it is *possible* to obtain such paragons of virtue and effectiveness considering the salaries usually available for parprofessionals in such programs, and the difficult nature of the job. Suprisingly, although it is not always possible to select persons with *all* of the characteristics of the ideal home visitor, it *is* possible to find a great many of these qualities among paraprofessionals who apply. Clearly, such qualities are not limited to those with college degrees or advanced training; many people with the qualifications necessary to do these jobs well are available if one takes the time and trouble to find them. When one remembers that the effectiveness of the program depends greatly upon the effort expended in selection of home visitors, such time can only be counted as well spent.

## TRAINING HOME VISITORS

Once selection has been accomplished, prospective home visitors, both with and without college degrees, need pre- and in-service training. Such training must include, as a minimum, the origins and impact of parent-child interaction styles, basic information in each of the program components mentioned earlier, and above all, communication, and personal interaction skills.

Once underway, most Home Start programs provided three weeks of in-service training which was usually a combination of group meetings, individual sessions with program trainers and other staff, films, role playing, readings, visits with other home visitors, and often classes in other agencies, and educational institutes. The pre-service and on-going in-service training for paraprofessionals working in the home must take into account that the nature of the job largely precludes home visitors learning by traditional informal channels, i.e., working side-by-side in the same office with professionals and more experienced paraprofessionals. The conditions of their job do not provide them opportunity to observe, model, and receive direct and indirect feedback from co-workers regarding performance. This makes close supervision, at least during the early stages of home visiting, of paramount importance.

Due to many different roles played by home visitors in Home Start programs as well as the extensive information and skills needed to work effectively, it should be stated categorically that no matter what the home visitor's background, training in home visiting is of considerable importance to program effectiveness. The training should be designed in-so-far as possible, *to take absolutely nothing for granted.* It is essential that the training program take into account as many different aspects of job performance as possible, and that it define *exactly* what the home visitor needs to do and what the goals and objectives are in each program component. It is important that trainers know *exactly* what home visitors need to *know* in order to do the job as defined by their agency. Finally, the training should be specifically designed to help the home visitor learn precisely those concepts and behaviors defined as needed to do the job effectively.

On the basis of the experiences with the Home Start demonstration programs, several factors regarding paraprofessional training have been observed. Generally, the most successful pre-service training has been that which at least, initially, is practical and concrete, and deals, as much as possible, with what-tos, how-tos, with realistic situations, and down-to-earth problems. This does not mean that there is no place for the whys, of theory, and research that underly procedures and practices; it does mean, at least initially, training that that stresses the concrete and practical is most effective.

No matter how extensive pre-service training may be, it is absolutely essential that there be provision for continued in-service training as a regular part of the week. Pre-service training must present the overall picture broadly. In in-service training important issues are discussed in depth, new areas presented and details filled in. Dr. Ann O'Keefe, former National Director of Home Start, suggests that such ongoing staff development, including planning time, should occupy at least 20% of staff time (the equivalent of about one day each week).

So important is training to the effective functioning of paraprofessionals as home visitors, and so widespread is the need for such training as programs throughout the country begin to incorporate aspects of the Home Start operation into their activities, that in 1975 HEW provided funding to establish Home Start Training Centers in six locations. These centers also serve approximately 30 families each so that trainees can actually make home visits as part of their training. The Home Start Training Center staff often travel widely to make follow-up visits to trainees' sites as well as to give short term (1-2 day) orientation and training workshops on the home-based concept.[7]

Parallel to the establishment of these training centers

[7] More information on these sites and their training can be obtained from Home Start, Administration for Children, Youth and Family, P.O. Box 1182, Washington, D.C 20013.

is an increasing interest in delineating the competencies that home visitors should have and establishing an objective and reliable means to assess and credential them. In 1978, the Child Development Consortium, (CDC) which had already developed a system for credentialing demonstrated competency in the staff of center-based child development programs, began a study of the feasibility of a similar CDA credential for those who deliver child development services to parents in their own homes. The development of such a system should greatly contribute to improving the training and preparation of home visitors as well as provide a means of formal recognition to those who can competently perform the complex task of home visitor.

## SUMMARY

Home Start, the many programs which preceded it, and the hundreds of home-based programs that have since begun, have been built on paraprofessionals who bring services directly to families in their own homes. In the last few years, the enormous growth of home-based (home visiting) programs has testified to the usefulness of this model in many different fields in addition to its appropriateness for providing a wide range of services to many different populations. The experiences of these programs, and especially those of the Home Start demonstration program itself, have made it indisputably clear that paraprofessionals can function effectively in home-based programs. The record clearly shows that with careful selection, training, supervision and support, the use of paraprofessionals in home-based programs is not only feasible, in terms of economy and quality of service, but may actually be the method of choice.

Many things have been learned. Home visiting is an enormously complex job requiring a great range of skills and competencies. Considerable training as well as particular personality traits are needed to do it well. Although the great variety of these programs makes it essential that the training be specific to the way the program actually operates, the author's experiences have also shown that there is a definable core of *competencies* and abilities fundamental to home visiting, per se, and a definable core of *needs* particular to those who work in homes. For this reason, it is impossible to overemphasize the importance to home visiting staff of having clear and continuing demonstrations of administrative support and understanding.

Through the Home Start demonstration, we have learned that paraprofessionals, given training and support, can be used effectively in a greater variety of ways than had previously been thought possible. Project administrators have started to learn what is necessary in terms of prerequisites and training to support these functions. In view of the fact that there is a growing need for efficient and effective ways to deliver many kinds of social services to different client groups, the findings of the Home Start demonstration regarding paraprofessionals in the home come as good news for all.

## REFERENCES

Bandura, A., & Walters, R.H., *Social learning and personality development*, New York: Holt Rinehart and Winston, 1963.

Gordon, I.J. *A home learning center approach to early stimulation*, Institute for Development of Human Resources, Gainesville, Fla., 1971 (Grant No. MH 16037-02).

Gray, S.W. & Klaus, R.A. *The early training project: The seventh-year report. Child Development*, 1970, *41.* 909-924.

Klaus, R.A. & Gray, S.W. *The Early Training Project for Disadvantaged Children: A Report After Five Years.*

Monographs of the Society for Research in Child Development, 1968, *33* (4), Serial No. 120

Levenstein, P. *Cognitive growth in preschoolers through verbal interaction with mothers.* American Journal of Orthopsychiatry, 1970, 40, 426-432.

Love J., et al. National Home Start Evaluation, Final Report; Findings and Implications, 1976. Available through Home Start, Administration For Children. Youth and Families, HEW, PO Box 1182, Washington, D.C. 20013.

Schaefer, E.S. *Progress Report: Intellectual Stimulation of Culturally deprived parents.* National Institute of Mental Health, 1968.

Weikart, D.P. et al. *Longitudinal results of the Ypsilanti Perry preschool project.* Ypsilanti, Mich.: High/-Scope Educational Research Foundation, 1970.

## ADDITIONAL READINGS

Giomer, B., Miller, J. O & Gray, S.W. *Intervention with mothers and young children: Study of intra-family effects.* Nashville, Tenn. DARCEE Demonstration and Research Center for Early Education, 1970.

*Guide for planning and operating home-based child development programs.* 1974. Available through: Home Start, Administration for Children, Youth and Families, Office of Human Development Services, Department of Health, Education and Welfare, P.O. Box 1182, Washington, D.C. 20013.

Hess, R.D., Shipman, V.C., Brophy, J.E. & Bear, R. M. *The cognitive environments of urban preschool children; Follow-up phase.* Chicago: University of Chicago Graduate School of Education, 1969.

*Home start and home start training centers brochure.* 1978. Brief description of Home Start. Lists locations of the six Home Start centers.

Karnes, M.B., Hodgins, A.S. & Teska, J.A. The impact of

at-home instruction by mothers on performance in the ameliorative preschool. In M.B. Karnes, *Research and Development Program on Preschool Disadvantaged Children: Final Report.* Washington, D.C.: U.S. Office of Education, 1969, 205-212.

Karnes, M.B., Teska, J.A., Hodgins, A.S. & Badger, E.D. *Educational Intervention at home by mothers of disadvantaged infants. Child Development,* 1970, *41,* 925-936.

Massoglia, T. *Early Childhood Education in the Home,* (with accompanying Instructor's Guide). New York: Delmar Publishers (Division of Litton Educational Publishing, Inc.), 1977.

O'Keefe, R. A. Home Start: Partnership with Parents. *Children Today,* Jan.-Feb. 1973, 2 (1), Available through: Home Start, Administration for Children, Youth and Families, Office of Human Development Services, Department of Health, Education and Welfare, P.O. Box 1182, Washington, D.C. 20013.

*Partners with parents: The home start experience with preschool children and their families,* 1978. Available through: Home Start, Administration for Children, Youth and Families, Office of Human Development Services, Department of Health, Education and Welfare, P.O. Box 1182, Washington, D.C 20013.

Schaefer, E.S. Need for Early and Continuing Education. In V.H. Denenberg (Ed.), *Education of the Infant and Young Child.* New York: Academic Press, 1970, 61-82.

# Indigenous Mental Health Paraprofessionals on an Indian Reservation[1]

Marvin W. Kahn,
*University of Arizona,*
Joseph Henry and Linda Lejero,
*Papago Psychological Service, Sells, Arizona*

Developing a meaningful mental health program that is relevant to a tribal Indian community's need and that will be acceptable to its people so that they will utilize it was the challenge in developing the Papago Psychological Service on the Papago Indian Reservation in southern

[1]The authors wish to acknowledge the following members of the Papago Psychological staff for their helpful comments regarding this chapter: Marian Antone, Lloyd Francisco, Darra Lorentine, Sharon Miguel, Richard Ramirez, Laura Smith, Kenneth Williams.

Arizona. The key elements in accomplishing this have been the development of paraprofessional Papago mental health technicians as the providers of service, and full policy and financial control by the Papago tribe.

Although Indians share many of the attributes of the culture of poverty (Lewis, 1959) with other American socio-economically deprived groups, the tribal Indians are distinctive in that they are still close to tribal origins, customs, and beliefs. They are people with their own language and, only relatively recently, removed from a hunter-gatherer, semi-nomadic style of life.

There has been less attention focused on the Native-American's economic and social plight than there has been for other disadvantaged minority groups. This is probably due to the relatively small number of Indians, their concentration on the reservations in a few remote areas, and their lack of militancy. There has also been little attention paid to Indians since an existing, if often inadequate, governmental welfare-caretaker system (Bureau of Indian Affairs and Indian Health Service) has been in existence for more than 146 years. Given the conditions of poverty, the accompanying factors of social disadvantage and low educational attainment that are faced by most of the Native-Americans, it seems reasonable to assume that severe and extensive mental health problems are at least as prevalent for them as is the case with the other disadvantaged groups that have been studied extensively.

It has been well established since the Hollingshead and Redlich (1958) study and Dohrenwend and Dohrenwend (1969) review that socioeconomically disadvantaged people (who most assuredly include American-Indians) have more mental health problems, and more severe mental health problems, than do the more socio-economically advantaged groups. Moreover, people in the lowest socio-economic stratum tend to receive the poorest services for these conditions. Particularly for individuals without "cushioning" sociocultural support, the circumstances of poverty, low economic, and social status create conditions of great stress. It is, therefore, not surprising to find a greater amount and degree of mental health problems with individuals from these circumstances. Moreover, several studies have shown (Imber et al., 1955; Kahn and Heiman, 1977) that when the services are provided and available, the lower socioeconomic minority people may not use them, or use them only briefly when they do. This lack of utilization of mental health services by the ethnic minority lower socio-economic persons seems to be due to value and cultural background differences between the usual white middle-class oriented professionals who are the providers of the services, and the recipients. Not only do the poor and minority group members have difficulty obtaining transportation to the clinic or hospital, but once there, they may feel strange and alien to the setting. Often, they find it very difficult to understand and thus trust the therapist and the methods being used. Self-disclosure, personal soul-searching, abstract concepts, and strange and different values about behavior may seem frightening, incomprehensible, and/or insulting. Although there certainly have been some notable exceptions to this pattern (Lerner, 1972; Goldstein, 1973), in most instances, the white, middle class providers appear to be a serious mismatch for the poor ethnic minority people with regard to mental health treatment.

To cope with these problems, mental health services provided by indigenous paraprofessionals from the community have been developed to provide services to socially disadvantaged people. Certainly, for a relatively traditional tribal Indian population which has its own language and deeply ingrained culture and value system, such an approach seemed appropriate. It was initiated with the understanding that the tribe itself believed there were mental health problems for which they needed special help. Consequently, they wanted a program to deal with such problems. Such a program, however, had to be compatible with their culture and value system and be conducted with full respect for their traditions and ways of doing things. Moreover, the program was to be truly theirs, both sponsored and run by their own people. The white professionals who played the roles in starting it had an obligation to rapidly turn it over to the Papagos themselves.

## DEVELOPING THE PAPAGO PSYCHOLOGICAL SERVICE

When this program was begun in 1969, mental health services to the Papago Indian Reservation consisted of a traveling mental health team from the Indian Health Service that visited the main village of the reservation for a few days once a year. Although they were eligible for services in the metropolitan areas of the state, an extremely small number of Papagos who lived on the reservation were served by these facilities.

In almost every area surveyed, massive mental health problems were indicated. In the schools, dropouts, poor attendance, poor achievement, drinking, and drug problems were among the most visible difficulties. The hospital saw many alcoholism-related problems, family difficulties, child neglect, neuroses, and psychoses. The tribal welfare and work programs were dealing with unemployed individuals, many of whom had severe drinking problems and related family difficulties. Law enforcement agencies dealt with many infractions of the law related to alcoholism, such as family arguments, fights, beatings, and child neglect, etc. The churches were involved in counseling many Indians regarding a variety of problems. The Bureau of Indian Affairs Social Services was besieged with all these and other problems. It was clear that the need for mental health services was present. Moreover, the tribe and the tribal officials were aware, concerned and supportive of a mental health facility which could help in this situation.

Alcoholism, broken homes, family and marital problems, child behavior difficulties, and a high suicide rate were the most obvious mental health problems at that time. Given an unemployment rate of more than 50%, and the history of the Indian cultural clash with the dominant western society, this is not surprising.

The Papago Psychological Service on the reservation was initially developed by a joint effort by the Papago tribe, the Clinical Psychology Program of the University of Arizona, and the Indian Health Service (Kahn and Delk, 1973).

## GAINING COMMUNITY ACCEPTANCE

The basic tenet in developing this service for the Papagos was that it would respect the traditional culture and would work within their ways of doing things. This included working cooperatively with the Papago medicine men, who are held in high respect by the tribal people. Many discussions were held with many Indian groups on the reservation on how best to develop services. A meeting also was held with a group of medicine men and the persons developing the clinic. In explaining the purpose of the clinic and how it would work, medicine men were invited to be consultants to the clinic for a professional fee. They also would be available to receive referrals from the clinic. Cases in which difficulties stemmed largely from the Papago cultural values were referred to the medicine men. Sometimes, medicine man healing was used as an additional service to the other psychological services as well. It was only when all elements of the tribe who were consulted had agreed to the clinic, that the tribe permitted it to begin.

## THE PAPAGO PEOPLE

In order to understand the crucial importance of having services provided by the indigenous people themselves, some background on the reservation environment, as well as the customs and beliefs of the Papago people is necessary. Although the Papago Indians are a tribe who have not been geographically displaced by white men, their living area has been greatly reduced. Nonetheless, the reservation consists of a large area of desert, about the size of the state of Connecticut. Since the Papagos were not displaced, their culture and living patterns are probably more intact and more traditional than some of the other tribes. Most Papagos now speak some English in addition to their own language; some of the older generation speak only Papago. Many of the homes are made of hand-fashioned, mud adobe block. They have dirt floors, and lack plumbing and electricity. In the larger villages, however, better housing and facilities are available to some Papagos.

The unemployment rate is more than 50%; welfare provides the main subsistence for a large number of people. There are two school systems on the reservation, one run by the Papago School Board, the other, maintained by the Bureau of Indian Affairs as boarding schools. A proportion of families living on the reservation have, at various periods, lived in other areas of the country, some in the larger cities. They have returned to a reservation because they found life in the cities and in the Anglo world undesirable. There is, then, a wide range of acculturation to the dominant society. It cannot be overlooked, however, that many are very traditional people, especially those who live in the outer villages.

In more traditional times, the parents would choose the marriage partners for the children and the couple would move in with the family unit of one or the other parent. Today, the couples make their own choice with regard to partners, but because of the unemployment situation and the scarcity of housing, the young couples still move in with one set of parents. It is not unusual for the marriages to essentially end after four or five years as the male may drift off into a pattern of drinking with other men and perhaps become involved with other women when drunk. The wife, now with several children, will stay with her mother and may find another man or men over the years. This is not to say, however, that there aren't many stable and long lasting marriages. But, the need for marriage and family counseling, however, is apparent.

Several Papago behavioral characteristics are different than those found in Western society. For the Papago, individual glory and besting others in competition is not regarded as very acceptable behavior. Thus, to outdo others in school or at work brings not reward, but social pressure and a threat of rejection. Papagos also maintain an emotional reserve and are not likely to openly express their feelings. It is very difficult for them to discuss personal and private matters with others. Sharing possessions is an important value among the people. When there is need, especially among the family members, the Papagos are expected to share what they have. This reduces the proclivity to work in order to save or even to conceptualize saving, since needy relatives can claim whatever a jobholder has gained. As these examples of behavioral characteristics indicate, many of the ways of the Papago are very different from those of middle-class whites and from the implied values in many of our current mental health techniques. Many of these patterns, however, are changing.

The traditional Papago belief is that illness is caused in two ways: by evildoers who cast spells on people, or by offending animals (often inadvertently) in their natural surroundings. The medicine man is the individual who has the power to diagnose the offending cause. It is of note that among the Papagos there is some specialization. One type of medicine man specializes in determining the cause of the disorder and another specializes in the cure. The diagnostic medicine man can determine the nature of the illness by blowing smoke over the patient and by waving sacred eagle feathers. The cure, or "Papago sing," is a ritual carried out by the other type of medicine man who uses various chants and sacred healing songs. He also will prescribe herbs, potions, dietary changes, and special rituals for the patient.

Offending certain desert animals, even unknowingly, causes certain types of human disorders. Offending a tarantula, for example, can cause pain in the neck; offending a turtle causes difficulty in walking. The horned toad causes pains in the joints and the deer, severe headaches. The owl is feared as the spirit of a person returning from the dead. It is interesting that persons who have committed suicide are said to belong to the devil.

These beliefs are deeply ingrained and rites stemming from them are practiced by many of the people. For others, the beliefs are weakly held. Some degree of belief, however, does seem to be present for almost everyone. The medicine men and their practices are held in deep respect, fear and awe by the people. Understanding of these traditional beliefs were an important cornerstone in working with the people within their culture.

## The Papago Mental Health Technicians

The language and the culture traits indicate that Papagos themselves had to be the central communicators in the helping process. The program started with a few white professionals, working closely with Papagos from other tribal programs, acting as translators, cultural links, and implementers of recommendations.

Full-time Papago paraprofessionals for the clinic were slowly added as funds became available. Each was trained in an apprentice fashion with professionals. Skills in interviewing, relating, assessing problem situations, and implementing treatment recommendations were taught to the paraprofessionals. Tutorial training with actual cases was supplemented by formal courses and lectures in staff meetings and, later, at training sessions and workshops as the program developed.

Selection of the individuals to become indigenous paraprofessionals mental health workers for this clinic was obviously a very important task. The following criteria for selection have gradually evolved and are used by the Papago selection committee.

1.  Prior educational attainment as such is not of major importance. It is necessary that the prospective trainee can understand enough English and concepts to follow some of the instructional opportunities. There are many perceptive, understanding, and self-taught individuals in disadvantaged groups who do not stay long in the formal school settings. A formal educational criterion was avoided because its use could eliminate some of the best candidates.

2.  Some minimal acculturation to the dominant society is desirable since the mental health technicians will be working with professional consultants, community agencies, and with techniques that require some acculturation for understanding. It is, however, more crucial that the trainees fully identify with their own group, rather than being oriented toward white middle-class society. In order for the program to be a truly indigenous one, the Papagos working with their own people as primary workers need to be in close touch with their own group in terms of their orientation, values, and commitment.

3.  The selected individuals should be responsive, warm, sensitive people capable of relating comfortably to a variety of individuals, basically interested in people and wanting to help and to be of service to them. Effective human relationships are the main vehicle through which mental health services are provided; they require providers who are interested, care, and can relate to others.

4. The individuals selected need to be free of any real major personal problems or disorders that might impair their effectiveness. But that is not to say that any indication of present or past difficulty would automatically exclude someone. No one is problem-free. The concern here is simply that no overwhelming, interfering problems are present.

## TRAINING PROCEDURES

The initial training with the first three Papago paraprofessionals was designed to develop skills in interviewing and relating to clients; this included some basic intervention techniques, starting with supportive counseling, and crisis intervention. This was accomplished on a one-to-one tutorial basis with the professionals who were available to the clinic. As the mental health workers became proficient in these areas, additional skills and techniques were added to their repertoire. Behavioral approaches and methods have been added in addition to marital, family and alcoholism counseling.

Training the paraprofessionals to administer and score intelligence tests has also been done. This is a very sensitive cultural area that requires knowledge of language and developing a comfortable relationship. With school attendance and achievement problems being substantial areas of difficulty on the reservation, culturally appropriate testing conditions and testers are important.

What methods and techniques the white, middle class trainers had to offer initially were those appropriate for a white, middle class clientele. These techniques, however, were not taught to be used unaltered. Rather, the methods and rationale were taught so that they could be adapted to the cultural and behavioral style of the Papagos. And, indeed, the way the Papago mental health workers interview, assess, or apply treatment succeed in being adaptive to the cultural group with which they are working. For instance, with Papagos it is considered aggressively intimate to look someone in the eye; further in discussion, one does not approach a problem directly. Rather, some lengthy talk about other things before gradually getting into the problem area is necessary if any meaningful communication is to take place.

In adopting group therapy to delinquent Papago adolescents, it was necessary to change some central features of this method in order to use it more effectively. Since discussing intimate personal problems is not a generally accepted thing to do among Papagos, this was even more delicate a matter with the teenagers. By keeping discussions, however, in somewhat abstract terms of dealing with problem situations, always in the third person so that individuals were not openly identified with their problem, it became possible to have very meaningful discussions of these feelings, situations, and solutions (Kahn, Lewis, and Galvez, 1974).

As the program has grown, new mental health technicians have been added. Their training has increasingly been carried out by the indigenous senior mental health technicians utilizing a similar tutorial model approach. As with the other groups, this is supplemented liberally with attendance at available workshops and conferences.

## THE SHIFT FROM PROFESSIONAL TO INDIGENOUS CONTROL

From a small beginning dominated by white professional direction, services, and training activities, the service steadily developed and increasingly expanded. Once the original group of three mental health workers had been trained and gained some experience, they took over the program and the training. The professional's role was reduced to that of consultant, which, while maintained through the years, has become less pronounced as it was needed less.

How this shift from white and professional direction to that of full control by the Papago, themselves, evolved is probably worthy of some comment since it is a goal apparently espoused by many programs, but one that is relatively infrequently achieved. In this case, it started with an initial, explicit commitment to make the program a truly Papago one. Good intentions, however, necessary as they are, are not sufficient. At the beginning stage, the conceptualization of how this truly Papago Clinic would happen was in terms of encouraging and developing Papago talent to enter training as professional mental health personnel, as social workers, psychologists, and psychiatrists,—a rather distant goal. But what could be done early, and what was probably decisive, was that full authority and financial control for the program could be given to the tribe. The Indian Health Service (the funding agency) agreed to this when the service was in operation for three years. The senior paraprofessional mental health worker became the clinic director with full authority for budget, hiring, and firing (including professional staff) and determining priorities. Given this authority and control, the Papagos clearly and rapidly demonstrated their desire to run their own program, and their ability to do it.

It was important that the professionals recognized the Papagos right and ability to do this; they displayed a willingness to work with them on their terms. The changeover was not without considerable initial anxiety on the part of the professionals or a period of confusion, some mistakes, and some vacilating between over-dependence and under-dependence on the consultants. But as the Papagos gained confidence and experience, they took hold very effectively and efficiently. The consultants' anxieties were considerably allayed by the generally good sense the Papagos showed in determining when they needed professional advice and when they did not. Support and encouragement from the consultants at that point was important, but so was allowing them to learn from experience. It became apparent, as things then developed, that the program could be run very effectively with relatively limited professional consultation. The role of the professional consultant in such a situation requires a rather different orientation than the usual role and is discussed in Kahn, et al., (1975).

Practical factors also undoubtedly played an influential role in this process as well. The basic professional in this case had neither a job nor career to protect in his continuing involvement with the program (the basic position was at a university), and a round trip to the reservation and back is 140 miles of desert. Moreover, the consulting fees when they were developed 1½ years after doing the initial work voluntarily, were deliberately kept under the going rates in town. Thus, some of the more blatant aspects of developing a career and a financially vested interest in the program were not operating to a great extent. One would suspect that factors that retard developing the independence of such indigenous programs often come down to those of vested interest in power and control, careers, jobs and security, as well as little faith in the trained indigenous personnel to do the job, and exaggerated fears of risking some sort of a clinical disaster by letting the indigenous personnel run the cases.

## CURRENT STATUS OF THE PAPAGO PSYCHOLOGY SERVICE

At the present time, the program consists of six mental health technicians. One of the more experienced technicians is serving as supervisor; another as assistant director of the program. The overall program director is also an experienced mental health technician.

In addition to the original mental health program, the Papago Psychology Service has also undertaken a special learning program for retarded Papago children. A day school for 11 retarded Papago children and a homebound program for 10 others is run. The staff consists of one certified teacher, one substitute teacher, three teacher aides, an administrator and a special coordinator, all of whom are Papago.

Another recent program expansion is the Infant Stimulation Project. This is designed for early detection of possibly handicapped children and for the initiation of preventive measures. The Papago woman who runs this program emphasizes training the parents to provide the proper attention and stimulation to maximize the development of their infants.

The major mental health program provides a variety of services emphasizing counseling for those experiencing family and marital difficulties, school children who are having academic difficulty or problems with truancy and attendance, and those with drug and alcohol difficulties. There is also further counseling and assessing for the courts in the process of adjudicating delinquency, and various other legal offenses. In all, a wide range of personal difficulties and problem behaviors are treated. Referrals come from many sources. Some clients are self-referred, others are referred from the schools, the courts, or the hospital and medical services.

Characteristics of cases seen over the most recent one year period are given in Table 1.

As can be seen from Table 1, more females utilize the service. The age range is extensive. The youngest patient was 15 months, the eldest, 101 years old. The bulk of cases, however, are adolescents and young adults. The hospital is the largest source of referrals, although schools and other tribal agencies are sources of most of the other cases. Some self-referrals do occur.

The range of emotional problems is great. Family marital is the single largest category, with depression next. Psychoses and neuroses are present in the case load. The relatively low alcoholism figure is due to the fact that many of the cases that are primarily presented as alcohol-

Table 1

Summary of Patient Characteristics, Referral Sources and
Presenting Problems of Cases Seen (N=307)

*Sex*

| | *Male* | | *Female* | |
|---|---|---|---|---|
| | N | % | N | % |
| | 131 | 43 | 176 | 57 |

*Age*

| *0-5* | | *6-12* | | *13-17* | | *18-35* | | *36+* | |
|---|---|---|---|---|---|---|---|---|---|
| N | % | N | % | N | % | N | % | N | % |
| 18 | 6 | 33 | 11 | 67 | 22 | 130 | 42 | 59 | 19 |

*Referral Sources*

| Indian Health Service Hospital | | *Schools* | | *Self* | | Law & Order Trial Court | | *Other** | |
|---|---|---|---|---|---|---|---|---|---|
| N | % | N | % | N | % | N | % | N | % |
| 153 | 50 | 61 | 20 | 31 | 10 | 31 | 10 | 31 | 10 |

*Presenting Problems*

| *Family/ Marital* | | *Depression* | | *Aggressive Anti-Social* | | Mental *Retar- dation* | | *School Behavior* | |
|---|---|---|---|---|---|---|---|---|---|
| N | % | N | % | N | % | N | % | N | % |
| 63 | 20 | 38 | 12 | 33 | 11 | 30 | 10 | 25 | 9 |

| *Psychotic or Neurotic* | | *Alcoholism* | | *Cognitive Testing* | | *Substance Abuse* | | *Child Abuse* | | *Other* | |
|---|---|---|---|---|---|---|---|---|---|---|---|
| N | % | N | % | N | % | N | % | N | % | | |
| 22 | 8 | 19 | 7 | 18 | 5 | 18 | 5 | 5 | 2 | 36 | 11 |

* Community Health Representatives, Bureau of Indian Affairs Social Service, Papago Legal Aid, Juvenile Court.

ism are dealt with by a separate tribal alcoholism program.

## Evaluation of Effectiveness

Not unlike most other mental health services throughout the country, no fully formal evaluation of effectiveness of the program has been done. The problems of doing such an evaluation adequately are well known. Even in the absence of formal evaluation, however, it can be said the Papago Psychology Service is reaching the people. The people are responding and utilizing it. The service is well supported by the community as witnessed by the increasing number of individuals who utilize it, by the expansion of the number of areas of service, and by the increases in staff and budget allotted to this program. This is a far cry from only eight years ago when no such services were available except for a few days a year, and during the same time when almost no Papagos used services that existed in the general community.

In many quarters, there was considerable skepticism initially regarding the possibility of establishing any kind of program in this situation, and particularly whether the Indians could master the role as mental health technicians, let alone to run and develop their own service. On those issues, the evidence is overwhelming that the skeptics were wrong.

There probably is another benefit to this program—the benefit to the paraprofessionals themselves. Through this work, they have developed a sense of mastery, success, and self-determination, which is not only personally satisfying but also a benefit for the whole Indian community.

### Implications and Generalizations for Other Programs

This mental health program was developed for a very

specialized situation, a tribal people, with their own language and customs, and a history different from many other minority groups. There is then a question of whether what has been learned and developed here can have applicability to other paraprofessional programs.

A partial answer to that has come from an opportunity to try this approach with another distant, but in many ways similar, ethnic group, Australian Aborigines. This program was carried out not for tribal Aborigines as had been originally intended, but for a community of Aborigines and Torres Strait Islanders who lived in a remote urban area, a situation more comparable to that of an urban ghetto than to that of the tribal group with which the program was originally developed. The basic professional consultant to the Papago program and one of the trained Papago mental health workers were the instructors in Australia for the Aborigines (Kahn, Henry and Cawte, 1976).

The factors the authors believe have been critical to the basic success of these programs and which would probably be very important in any program for ethnic minority, lower socio-economic people are these:

1. First and foremost that the ethnic minority group being served need to have full control of their program to make the basic decisions with regard to what kind of services and what kind of priorities they, as a community, wish to have.

2. From that position, the indigenous authority system chooses whom they wish to work for them. Thus, they can develop their own people to provide the services and work toward their goals.

3. Selection of the paraprofessionals should be made by indigenous people themselves, bearing in mind criteria that have proved useful in other programs. The paraprofessionals that will be accepted by the community need to represent their values and culture. A tempting mistake is to pick paraprofession-

als on the bases of the best western education and ability to communicate well with the professionals, while neglecting the crucial aspects of shared values and identify with the indigenous community.

4.  The paraprofessionals chosen for the program need systematic training in basic relationships and mental health skills. It is necessary that they have the indigenous qualifications above, but without considerable orientation and skill training they are not prepared to function adequately. The training approach is very important. Some of the general aspects of it are reported in Kahn, Henry, and Cawte (1976).

    The training, however, is to provide a basic framework in methods and skills that indigenous people can adapt to their own culture and situation. Many of the methods developed for middle-class clientele can be adapted to other cultures, but others are quite inappropriate.

5.  In the early formative stages respect for the people's culture, ability, and right to develop their own program on their own terms, with support and encouragement along these lines, is important.

6.  Positive experience in training, encourages paraprofessionals to seek additional learning experiences and establishes the ground work for comfortable lasting relationships with professional consultants.

7.  Lastly, the sense of achievement, developing self-confidence, and self-respect engendered by their new knowledge, status, and by their own sense of effectiveness brings forth a great deal of personal growth. It also increases maturity. That kind of change and development has, for some, led to involvement in broader and, in some ways, more im-

portant roles with their people. This should be expected and encouraged.

The authors have been encouraged by the results of these programs. There are some aspects of them which are unique to the culture and the situations; there are also some general principles that seem to underlie what is being done, these are: respect for the people's culture and ways, allowing indigenous people to have full control and authority over programs, and having as the paraprofessionals, well trained representatives of the group they serve. These are factors the authors believe are basic and should have applicability to a wide variety of paraprofessional programs.

## REFERENCES

Dohrenwend, B. P. & Dohrenwend, B. S. *Social status and psychological disorders: A causal inquiry.* New York: Wiley, 1969.

Goldstein, A. P. *Structured learning therapy: Toward a psychotherapy for the poor.* New York: Academic Press, 1973.

Hollingshead, A. B. & Redlich, F. C. *Social class and mental illness.* New York: Wiley, 1958.

Imber, S. D., Nash, E. H., & Stone, A. R. Social class and duration of psychotherapy. *Journal of Clinical Psychology,* 1955, *11,* 281-284.

Kahn, M. W. & Delk, J. L. Developing a community mental health clinic on the Papago Indian reservation. *International Journal of Social Psychiatry,* 1973, *19,* 299-306.

Kahn, M. W. & Heiman, E. Factors associated with length of treatment in a barrio-neighborhood mental health service. *International Journal of Social Psychiatry,* 1978, *24,* 259-262.

Kahn, M. W., Henry, J. and Cawte, J. E. Mental health services by and for Australian Aborigines. *Aus-*

*tralian and New Zealand Journal of Psychiatry, 1976, 10,* 221-228.

Kahn, M. W., Kennedy, E. V. & Cawte, J. E. Mental health services by and for Aborigines and Islanders: A follow-up report. *Australian and New Zealand Journal of Psychiatry,* 1978, (March issue).

Kahn, M. W. Lewis, J. & Galvez, E. An evaluation of a group therapy procedure with reservation adolescent indians. *Psychotherapy: Theory and Practice,* 1974, *11,* 241-244.

Kahn, M. W., Williams, C., Galvez, E., et al. The Papago psychology service: A community mental health program on an American Indian reservation. *American Journal of Community Psychology,* 1975, *3,* 81-87.

Lerner, B. *Therapy in the ghetto: Political impotence and personal disintegration.* Baltimore: Johns Hopkins University Press, 1972.

Lewis, O. *Five families: Mexican case studies in the culture of poverty.* New York: Basic Books, 1959.

# A University-Based New Careers Program

Mary R. Harvey and Lynn E. Passy
*School of Community Service and Public Affairs,*
*University of Oregon*

Commitment to social reform, knowledge of the political constraints affecting human service delivery, and competence to do community development are the most valued educational outcomes of the University of Oregon's New Careers in Mental Health (NCMH) program.[1]

[1] The New Careers in Mental Health program was supported by a National Institute of Mental Health training grant (5 T41 MH13606-01, -02, -03, -04, and -05; 1973-1978). New Careers is located in the University of Oregon's School of Community Service and Public Affairs, an interdisciplinary undergraduate and professional school providing upper-division and graduate preparation for mental health, human service and public management careers. Although Federal funding has terminated, portions of the program continue to operate.

One of the few paraprofessional development programs to be located at a university, NCMH instituted educational services and policies to expand paraprofessional participation in higher education and has involved New Careerists in the institutional change process. Participants in the program were non-credentialed, career-oriented workers from a wide variety of local human service agencies. New Careers developed for these participants interdisciplinary and largely field-based education programs at both the associate (community college) and bachelor (university) levels. In both programs, New Careerists used the educational setting of a core seminar to examine community needs and design new service possibilities. In the process, they conducted an independent review of local services and formed, with one another, a social support group for self-conscious career decision making.

Program accomplishments have been impressive. Since 1973, a total of 87 New Careerists from 21 mental health/human service agencies participated. Most realized significant academic and career achievements. Virtually all experimented with new service roles and developed or broadened their community problem-solving, advocacy, and change-agent skills (Harvey and Passy, 1975). Manpower policies in participating agencies have been reshaped to ensure paraprofessionals access to higher education and to allow for competence-based career mobility. The educational innovations developed by New Careers gained community and campus support and are now funded primarily with local rather than grant dollars. Of most important interest, new service programs have been generated and paraprofessional competence to perform leadership roles has been affirmed (Harvey, 1976).

Overall, the New Careers grant has demonstrated that innovations in higher education can have a positive impact on the quality of local services and on the competence of local manpower. Program experience documented the difficulties inherent in tapping this potential and in overcoming the university's resistance to change (Harvey and Passy, 1977). The purpose of this article is to look at the role of higher education in paraprofessional development. The authors will review how a university-based New Careers program—a program with a social reform focus—cultivated the university as a base for paraprofessional impact. The article begins by describing program development themes in NCMH. Next, it considers how student and agency diversity, as well as particular educational innovations, have combined to produce university reform at one level and university impact on local service delivery and manpower issues at another. Finally, the article discusses lessons learned and issues raised during the course of the program.

## PROGRAM THEMES

There are five themes that provide a conceptual framework for program development in NCMH.

1.  *Paraprofessionals can help meet unmet human needs.* Pearl and Riessman (1965) were among the first to associate New Careers models of paraprofessional development with the public's need for improved services. In this view, non-credentialed workers, indigenous to the community, can do more than serve as auxiliaries to professionals in traditional practice. Some of the qualities they can bring to bear on social reform are personal investment in change, skills and knowledge underrepresented in the professional community, as well as untapped reserves of problem-solving and leadership ability. These are the qualities of paraprofessionals that need emphasis and cultivation if the improvements in mental health service envi-

sioned by the community health movement are to
be realized (Kelly, Snowden, and Muñoz, 1977).
Leadership in the creation and expansion of community care programs, involvement in the design
and delivery of preventive rather than therapeutic
or rehabilitative services, and community development to empower under- and/or poorly-served
populations remain critical needs. Paraprofessionals can, and should, address these needs.

2.  *Maximizing paraprofessional contribution requires the restructuring of human service work.*
Paraprofessionals do not exist in a vacuum. They
are members of complex agencies with more or less
entrenched service delivery structures. The onus
is on them to establish their legitimacy, when
legitimacy is all-too-easily and too often equated
with competence to perform traditional roles. If
paraprofessional efforts to acquire new and needed
stature are to be realized in service improvements,
then agency practices and professional as well as
paraprofessional roles must be reassessed. Finally,
if maximum contribution is to be expected, paraprofessionals require policies that provide a full
array of career options. Career ladders must offer
multiple levels of entry and allow for competence-
based advancement. On-going access to higher
education and continued training must be guaranteed.

3.  *Higher education is a necessary partner in paraprofessional development.* The mental health/hu-
man service field is a highly credentialed one.
Unless higher education extends its resources to
the already employed, it will help to lock paraprofessionals into dead-end positions by continuing to provide newly credentialed middle class
manpower to be promoted over them. In short,
higher education offers the credentials that paraprofessionals need as a base for career options.

330 PARAPROFESSIONALS IN THE HUMAN SERVICES

More importantly, higher education can—if it will —offer independent settings in which paraprofessionals can review on-going experience and gain knowledge, skills, and abilities essential to improved practice.

4. *Paraprofessionals are key resources for one another's growth and impact.* Paraprofessionals typically face numerous barriers to professional and personal growth. In agencies, they too often work at the bottom of career systems and are regarded by their professional colleagues as having limited capability and questionable legitimacy. In higher education, they represent a marginal student group—i.e., older, working, with family responsibilities and financial obligations—a group whose academic needs and career interests receive little attention. The combination of these circumstances can easily undermine self-esteem and thwart risk-taking competence. Interaction with, and social support from, others who share similar stresses and have similar aspirations can make the difference between perseverance and defeat for New Careerists. Study groups, cooperative babysitting, and tutorial assistance become supports to personal growth that New Careerists can extend to one another. Once organized, paraprofessionals can constitute themselves into a political force for securing needed changes in education, work, and service. Through contact with one another, individual needs are recognized as group needs and action can be taken to secure appropriate resources.

5. *An ecology exists among the various settings in which paraprofessionals are active.* Recently, Kelly (1977) extended his ecological concepts to social support systems, noting that individual accomplishment cannot be considered apart from the social settings in which that individual partici-

pates. The analysis applies to paraprofessional development programs. Work, school, home, and community interact to define the quality of environmental supports available to paraprofessionals seeking new career opportunities and influence. Personal stress can erode interest in higher education, and continued disregard in the work setting can contribute to personal stress. Similarly, success in higher education and contact with a widening circle of colleagues and peers can help build a new sense of self and encourage faith in one's own ability to make a genuine contribution.

Together, these five themes imply that a New Careers program oriented to social change must seek institutional reform of service, manpower, and educational practices and simultaneously develop in work, school, and home environments reciprocal supports to paraprofessional growth. Moreover, New Careerists must be involved in both activities.

## Program Approaches

In NCMH, two approaches seem to have yielded this supportive ecology. The first is the decision to enroll as many paraprofessionals from as many local agencies as possible. The second is the effort to build university and community college services to address personal and career as well as academic concerns of New Careerists. These approaches are discussed in the sections that follow.

### New Careerists: Diverse Students from Multiple Agencies

An evolving characteristic of NCMH has been the diversity of its participants. Over the course of the project, 21 agencies operating 33 distinct service programs have participated. These programs differ with respect to administration, services provided, and target populations. They differ also in terms of size, funding level, and organizational stability. New Careerists have come from large, relatively well-established state and county agencies, and from small community action programs. Some agencies have had a stable financial base while others have had to depend on uncertain levels of support from several sources.

Diversity is also evident in the patterns of paraprofessional utilization characterizing the New Careers participant agencies. Some have used paraprofessionals reluctantly and/or in carefully prescribed, tangential roles. Others have employed paraprofessionals almost exclusively, utilizing them at all levels in order to manage limited budgets and marginal agency existence. Still others have been experimental with both professional and paraprofessional roles allowing service needs and individual staff competence to guide the arrangement of work roles.

New Careerists entering the program from these varied settings differ not only in positions held and roles played but also in the kind and clarity of education and career goals prompting their entry into New Careers. Most enter to secure credentials that will facilitate upward mobility within the employing agency. Some, however, hope to improve competencies relevant to current positions and have no particular interest in advancement. Others are looking for ways to move into different roles or settings as well as for new career directions.

Agency and student diversity has presented a constant challenge to the program—straining program resources and, at times, obscuring program direction. Nevertheless, each year the decision to reach out to paraprofessionals playing varied roles in varied settings has been renewed.

The authors see a three-fold advantage to agency and student diversity. First, it enables New Careerists to organize for community benefit and interpersonal support. Since 1973, New Careerists have constituted perhaps the only group of local service practitioners meeting across agency lines on a weekly basis. By using the New Careers core seminar as a setting in which to share information about different client groups, community needs and problem-solving approaches, they have formed a social network for community action and personal growth. New Careerists have developed with one another formal and informal ways of expediting multi-agency service to individual clients. They have helped each other think through and obtain program modifications in participating agencies. New Careerists have secured, for example, expansion of a community health education office and created a sex education program for adult and adolescent retardates. Their dialogue has affirmed each other's ability to identify community needs and to design important alternatives. They have helped one another develop the courage needed to act as advocates of change.

Second, the inclusion of New Careerists from many settings has enabled the program to gather persuasive evidence for educational reform. Community colleges and universities are experiencing a loss of students and a concommitent loss of financial and human resources. By reaching out to a diverse New Careers population, the program has been able to identify for the community college and the university a new and potentially expanding student population and to demonstrate that educational resources can be developed to attract and serve these students. Without the persuasive power of sufficient numbers, New Careers educational programs would have little chance of surviving beyond federal funding.

Finally, involvement with diverse agencies and workers gives direction and substance to educational content. It enables us at the university to study the applicability of a generalist model of human service education, and, in the process, facilitate ongoing review of service needs and service modalities. The New Careers participant agencies

constitute a good sample of community service bureau-
cracies in action. Their approaches to service delivery
and manpower utilization can be compared, and different
service modalities (e.g., prevention, treatment, community development) can be contrasted. Program participants have a unique opportunity for studying the
political and economic events that influence service delivery as well as an opportunity to analyze these events
independently of agency interpretation and professional
traditions. Faculty are challenged to establish and maintain the relevance of a generalist model to events which
most concern agencies and New Careerists.

## Educational Reforms Required for New Careers Development

In a university-based New Careers program, educational innovation is the main vehicle for developing paraprofessional competence and creating change in local
service agencies (Passy, 1976). NCMH has developed at
both the community college and university educational
programs that provide needed access, relevant curriculum, and increased opportunity for contractual study
and field-based learning. Policy reforms secured in participating agencies (e.g., improved career ladders and
education release-time guarantees) ensure participation
and make possible career benefits, while the education
provided encourages agency and New Careerist experimentation with new service roles.

Access to higher education is first of all enhanced by
the existence of a visible educational resource center such
as the NCMH program has become. Here, New Careerists
can get academic advising tailored to their work situation
and career direction, help in charting feasible degree programs, information about specific courses, instructors
and course-challenge opportunities, plus knowledge of social, recreational, and educational resources available on
campus. Whereas non-working students may have the

time and energy to cull out these supports, New Career-sits do not and cannot. Their academic progress can be stymied unless appropriate support services exist.

New Careers has also improved access by helping to re-structure academic delivery at both the community college and university. The New Careers Academic Delivery System, Figure 1, incorporates site-delivered core seminars and credits for field-based learning with other site-delivered and on-campus course options. The model enables New Careerists to combine full-time work with full-time education and make normal progress towards desired degrees, Figure 2.

Figure 1. The New Careers in Mental Health "Academic Delivery System."

| A. WORK-BASED EDUCATION, e.g., Supervised Field, Independent Study, In-Service Training | B. SITE-DELIVERED CORE SEMINARS, e.g., New Careers Philosophy, Introduction to Commnity Mental Health, Program Development and Evaluation |
|---|---|
| C. SITE-DELIVERED COURSEWORK (other than core), e.g., English Composition, Biological Sciences, Sociology, etc. | D. CAMPUS-BASED COURSEWORK, e.g., Economics, Special Education, Art |

With respect to this design, the following highlights should be noted:

1. The credits and curriculum associated with Cell A stem entirely from on-the-job performance and work-based learning experiences. They involve virtually no use of released time.

2. The credits and curriculum associated with Cells B

and C involve minimal use of released time and provide maximized educational accessibility.

3. The credits and curriculum associated with Cell D involve use of released time for travel to and from, as well as participation in, campus-based education.

Paraprofessional access to higher education is only partially accomplished through reform of university and community college programs and traditions. Involvement in degree-oriented programs must also be supported by agency policy and attitude. Needed are release-time policies that permit enrollment without loss of pay, and active encouragement by professionals who value such options. To encourage the creation of such policies, NCMH requires that agencies, rather than individuals, apply for New Careers participation. Application forms ask that agencies articulate policies which support paraprofessional involvement and provide career ladder incentives to participation. When no such policies exist, New Careers faculty collaborate with agency administrators in their design. To date, all New Careers agencies have created release-time policies; 20 of them have continued and/or expanded these to include professional and clerical staff as well.

With the development of release-time policies, New Careers agencies have begun to identify accredited New Careers coursework as a legitimate vehicle for in-service training. Agency training monies have been made available for tuition, and some New Careerists have secured career advancements largely because of academic achievements realized in New Careers.

*Curriculum: Stress on community problem solving.* Paraprofessional development programs that fail to address the political and psychological circumstances of paraprofessionals can unwittingly encourage complacency, and foster uncritical acceptance of traditional service values. Lacking credentials, stature, and economic parity, paraprofessionals are often in positions of limited power and legitimacy. Their self-esteem can be severely

Figure 2. New Careers as an alternative route to a credential.

| Aide | New Careerist | Traditional College Student |
|---|---|---|
| Works full time. | Works full time. | Works part time, if at all. |
| Uses release time for in-service. | Uses release time for education on campus. | Spends most of time on campus or nearby. |
| Enrolls in accredited education as the opportunity arises, if at all. | Enrolls in NC-designed education program 4 terms per year (Fall, Winter, Spring and Summer). | Enrolls in traditional education program on campus 3 terms per year (Fall, Winter and Spring). |
| May enroll each term in a probable maximum of between 3 and 6 credit hours, or D type*. | Is able to enroll each term in 10-13 credit hours: 4-Cell A; 3-Cell B; 3-Cell C; and 3-6-Cell D type*. | Enrolls in an average of 15 credit hours each term all (or by far the majority) of Cell D Experiences*. |
| Is able to complete between 12 and 15 credits of questionable degree applicability per year. | Is able to complete between 40 and 52 credit hours per year at the above rate. | Typically completes 45 credit hours per acaemic year at the above rate. |
| Probably can't get a degree, or will | Is able to complete a 4-year degree in | Is able to complete a 4-year degree program |
| take 10+ years doing so at the above rate. | 3-4 years at this rate (186 hours are typically required). | in 4 years at this rate. |
| Is educated in 2 settings (work & campus) yet is unable to gain academic or career mobility from such experience. | Is educated in 2 settings (work & campus and is able to apply both sets of experience to degree career mobility. | Is educated in 1 setting (campus) and is able to utilize credential to obtain professional-level employment. |

*See Figure 1.

undermined, and the pressure to mold career aspirations around established agency patterns can be extreme.

To counter such possibilities, the NCMH curriculum emphasizes social and political awareness and encourages community activism. The goal is to foster a strong sense of accountability for quality service, and to encourage leadership and risk-taking skills necessary to public advocacy. At the community college, New Careers education focuses on six core courses which analyze social and political issues influencing the context, design, and direction of public service, Table 1. Theory-practice integration seminars at the School of Community Service and Public Affairs (CSPA) allow upper division New Careerists to deepen their study of these same issues. In both settings, the issues raised are examined in light of New Careerists' work experiences.

Whether at the community college or at CSPA, the New Careers seminar functions as a setting for community problem solving. Individually or in groups, New Careerists conduct projects using social analysis and action skills to address local problems. For example, in the seminar titled, "Political and Economic Foundations of Community Service," focus is on political processes that shape community needs and control public service funding and programming patterns. Discussions, guest lectures, and simulated games of power politics introduce the importance of competencies such as client advocacy, planning, and coalition building. New Careerists demonstrate their acquisition of these competencies in individualistic ways in term projects. One analyzes local implications of federal legislation vis-a-vis services to the trainable mentally retarded. Another develops a proposal for restructuring a community education service, identifying the political issues which the proposal faces en route through various segments of county bureaucracy. Feedback and dialogue about these projects helps New Careerists use class effort for impact. In these instances, the first New Careerist presented her work to a local service planning board. The second secured agency endorsement of her plan to expand service.

*Contractual study and field-based learning.* Direct translation of education into action, as well as support for experimentation with new paraprofessional roles, has been accomplished through the program's expansion of contractual study and field-based learning opportunities. Both are educational innovations essential to university support of paraprofessional development.

First, *contractual study.* The learning contract is a process of educational planning which demands accountability from, and negotiation by, both students and faculty. Students—i.e., New Careerists—assert learning goals, propose educational activities, identify learning resources, and suggest criteria for evaluation. Faculty facilitate this process, negotiate content and ensure that academic standards are met. The use of learning contracts enhances university responsiveness to individual learning needs, ensures credibility, sanctions education that occurs in community settings, and markedly expands the academic options of work-based adults. In NCMH, learning contracts have been developed for short-term reading and conference or special projects and, for a few New Careerists, have outlined entire degree programs.

Second, *field-based learning.* The learning contract process is also used to design field-based learning in NCMH. Here, agency experimentation with new paraprofessional roles and new professional/paraprofessional relationships is encouraged. The agency is designated a learning environment. Agency supervisor, New Careers faculty, and New Careerist negotiate a contract in which an identified community mental health role (valued by the program and relevant to community need and agency service possibilities) is introduced. New Careers faculty ensure that a theoretical framework guides role exploration and accredit agreed-upon learning projects.

By completing these projects under both agency and

university supervision, the New Careerist not only acquires new competencies but also studies the relevance of these competencies to specific community needs and particular work activities. By offering academic credit and technical assistance, the program provides agencies with incentive for innovation and creates a context for experimentation. The agency supervisor takes on an advocate and support role vis-à-vis the New Careerist, becoming a key participant in the design of new service roles. The New Careerist is moved into a negotiating role with both faculty and agency professionals. Faculty roles are reshaped and refocused toward greater community involvement. The process ensures consideration of community need in designing accredited learning and/or specified work activities. Faculty become resources to activities valued by the community and the agency is defined as a valid learning environment. Overall, the process affirms the maturity and contribution of the paraprofessional by identifying the New Careerist as an active participant in both educational planning and service design.

## Conclusions and Implications

What are the key lessons of the New Careers program at the University of Oregon? First and primarily, we have learned that the university can provide a solid base for New Careers. It can: 1) offer academic credit and degrees needed for career advancement; 2) offer relevant coursework; 3) accommodate diverse students, 4) link education across disciplinary lines; and 5) provide a setting in which to study social events, develop professional skills, and refine professional values. In addition, it can reach out to new students and provide impetus for change in community colleges and local agencies. The university has critical resources and enormous potential in relation to New Careers program development.

The university, however, does not always do what it can do. Despite its potential, the university is reluctant to pursue educational directions valued by New Careers. Liberal Arts education and classroom-based learning continue to be the first priority. Faculty roles that gain support are entrepreneurial in nature and remote from community concerns. The application of knowledge is not yet as valued as the genesis of knowledge. These traditions not only support university distance from the local community but also limit faculty contribution. Thus, the second lesson of NCMH is that institutional reform of the university is a necessary element of paraprofessional development programming. New admission policies and advising practices must invite real participation by working adults. Interdisciplinary content must characterize undergraduate human service career education, and such education must be better understood and valued. Prevailing views of appropriate educational methods and settings must be broadened. In particular, contractual study, the use of community settings as learning environments, and educational techniques that enhance theory-practice integration must be expanded and gain legitimacy. Most important, new faculty roles and new faculty-community relationships must receive institutional support and affirmation.

The third lesson of NCMH is that paraprofessional development programs can be successful catalysts for university reform. The New Careers program at the University of Oregon has sought and secured needed change. This success can be attributed to several causes. First, the educational changes sought by NCMH have validity in their own right. Students, other than New Careerists need diverse learning opportunities, and both faculty and community can benefit from broadened collaboration. There are in both community and campus allies for university reform. Second, the New Careers program has, from the onset, made institutional reform a central theme, actively seeking opportunities for influence on the larger academic system. Allies for change may exist within the university, but leadership for change is missing. Paraprofessional development efforts must provide it. Third, New Careerists have been actively involved in the definition of needed changes and in the political and educational process of securing them. New Careerist involvement gives energy and direction to the change process. Finally, the experimental nature of the NCMH program has provided a rationale and context for testing and establishing the legitimacy of new faculty roles. An experimental context minimizes institutional risk until the validity of particular innovations has been demonstrated.

In the end, the best argument for basing a New Careers program in the university is that higher education continues to be a necessary partner in any paraprofessional development effort that values social reform. The university can be a willing or reluctant partner in that effort. If New Careers programs identify allies within the university, mobilize community pressure for university change, and provide New Careerists with a base for full involvement, then the university can offer more than academic credentials and can become for New Careerists a vital setting for personal and professional growth.

## REFERENCES

Harvey, M. R. New Careerists: Paraprofessionals as resources for improving services. In James G. Kelly (Chair), *New Careers in community mental health: The impact of paraprofessionals on the quality of service delivery.* Symposium presented at the meeting of the Western Psychological Association, Los Angeles, April, 1976.

Harvey, M. R. & Passy, L. E. Paraprofessional development in New Careers in Mental Health. In James G. Kelly (Chair), *Undergraduate education for profes-*

*sional careers: An Oregon story*. Symposium presented at the meeting of the American Psychological Association, Chicago, August, 1975.

Harvery, M. R. & Passy, L. E. New Careers: The creative use of marginality. *Journal of Alternative Human Services, (forthcoming)*.

Kelly, J. G. The ecology of social support systems: Footnotes to a theory. In Julian Rappaport (Chair), *Toward an understanding of natural helping systems*. Symposium presented at the meeting of the American Psychological Association, San Francisco, August, 1977.

Kelly, J. G., Snowden, L. R. & Muñoz, R. F. Social and community interventions. *Annual Review of Psychology*, 1977, *28*, 323-61.

Passy, L. E. Creating an educational support system for New Careers. In James G. Kelly (Chair), *New Careers in community mental health: The impact of paraprofessionals on the quality of service delivery.*Symposium presented at the meeting of the Western Psychological Association, Los Angeles, April, 1976.

Pearl, A. and Riessman, R. *New Careers for the Poor*. New York: MacMillan Publishing Co., Inc., 1965.

# IV. AN OVERVIEW

# Reality, Rhetoric and the Paraprofessional: A Concluding Note

Morton O. Wagenfeld and Stanley S. Robin,
*Western Michigan University*

This volume has dealt with paraprofessionals in the human services. A term that is frequently used to describe this phenomenon is the "paraprofessional movement." It seems appropriate to characterize it in this way because it displays the characteristics associated with a social movement: leaders, followers, and ideology, and a set of goals (cf. Heberle, 1951; Killian and Turner, 1972, McPherson, 1973; Roberts and Kloss, 1974). As with any social movement that seeks to bring about changes in society as a whole or some segment of it, the paraprofessional movement has generated a great deal of controversy. Indeed, it is unlikely that any innovation in human

347

services delivery has evoked as much debate. Have paraprofessionals revolutionized and revitalized the delivery of human services or are they some anachronism of the ameliorative *zeitgeist* of the 1960s? The contributors to this volume were chosen both for their expertise in particular fields and in the belief that their articles would reflect a balanced diversity of perspectives and opinions. That there is diversity of opinion about the global success of the movement and its future is evident: the assessments are antipodal.

Franklyn Arnhoff, who was involved in the development of manpower and training programs while at NIMH, offers a very gloomy picture of the fate of paraprofessionalism in this volume:

> In a period of a little over a decade, the new careers-paraprofessional movement has moved from a zenith of governmental and professional development and active promulgation to a nadir of inactivity and almost to obscurity.

Alan Gartner, one of the contemporary leaders in paraprofessional training and education, although admitting that they are no longer "media sexy" argues that "far from fading" paraprofessionals are so much a part of the fabric of human services they are no longer separable. He predicts a bright and extensive future for the paraprofessional.

Arthur Pearl, who was "present at the Creation," offers still another view. For Pearl, the movement was a success, but there are virtually no new New Careers programs left. Moreover, little has changed in the institutions that were supposed to be changed by the New Careers approach.

How does one go about reconciling these seemingly

irreconcilable positions? One beginning is a recognition that the movement arose from diverse sources with multiple purposes and was suffused with the romantic ideology that was present in the early and mid 1960s. Basically, this ideology held that it was possible to change the structure of society and to ameliorate some of the more pernicious social problems (e.g., racism, mental disorders, poverty) through massive infusions of federal funds. Some of the more notable products of this era were VISTA; Peace Corps; Model Cities; and, to a certain extent, Community Mental Health. Partly growing out of this ideology, the purposes for which the paraprofessionals were created often became unclear, contradictory, and unrealistic.

In the early years of the New Frontier and the War on Poverty, large numbers of the poor were hired to fill certain low level positions. The tradition of this type of subprofessional or paraprofessional was certainly not new: for some time there had been various categories of aides in education, health care, and mental health. The prevailing view, as Pearl points out so well, was that incumbents or beneficiaries of these positions were poor because they were the victims of accumulated environmental and structural deficits. Providing them with jobs would be a form of compensatory justice.

In their seminal *New Careers for the Poor* (1965), Pearl and Riessman rejected this "deficit theory" and argued, instead, that poverty was the result of a lack of opportunities and that paraprofessional programs should go beyond their previously limited scope and become instruments of structural change. The New Careers approach would accomplish three things. First, it would provide dignified and significant employment for the poor. Second, it would also help to ameliorate some of the glaring defects in the human services delivery system. Finally, by providing opportunity structures or career ladders, the poor who were hired as paraprofessionals could become upwardly mobile. In a sense, the early paraprofessional efforts at creating low-level employment for the poor—based on a simple deficit model—were unitary in purpose and relatively straightforward. The multipurpose approach advocated by Pearl and Riessman and, later, widely adopted, contained the potential for problems in assessment. Does one judge the success of the movement in terms of the number of jobs created, the extent to which the defects in the human services delivery system had been altered, the amount of upward mobility that had taken place, or some combination of these?

Riley (Note 1), in reviewing the literature on paraprofessionals, has observed that several additional functions were proposed for them: paraprofessionals would act as bridgemen and activists. Due to the fact that they would (presumably) be drawn from the ranks of the poor and populations who were traditional recipients of the health and human services, they would better understand the problems and be better able to act as "sociocultural bridges" between these clients and the largely white, middle-class professionals. This relates to Pearl and Riessman's notion of "humanizing" the human services. Additionally, because they were "of the poor," the paraprofessionals would be more sensitive to the injustices and outrages of the system and be more militant about changing it.

The authors maintain that assessing the global effectiveness of the paraprofessional movement has been made difficult by the diversity of purposes and roles for which the paraprofessionals were created. It is not surprising, then, that evaluating specific training programs is rather difficult. Blanton and Alley have decried the lack of well-planned, well-used, and well-implemented evaluations of paraprofessional programs. Part of the difficulty, they note correctly, lies in the fact that the evaluation process is also a political process. To evaluate any program is to—at least in principle—commit oneself to a decision regarding continuation or termination. For paraprofessionals, the political process has an additional salience because training programs in the human services have been designed to ameliorate issues with high political visibility seen as alcoholism, drug addiction, poverty, inadequate education, crime, and mental disorder. As the front-line troops in this massive battle, paraprofessionals were invested with a certain romantic aura. The net effect was to stifle or, at best, inhibit, critical evaluation as somehow "anti-humanitarian." The programs were "right" in some ultimate moral sense; ideological considerations should take precedence over programmatic goals, research findings, or economic cost/benefit ratings.

The reports and assessments of paraprofessional programs in specific areas reflect the same inconsistencies as do the earlier articles by Arnhoff, Gartner, Pearl, and Haskell. Elovson, Kahn et al., Schneidmuhl et al., and Gartner report successful, efficient paraprofessional programs. Harvey and Passy and Scott describe generally successful paraprofessional programs but both accounts detail ways in which the training and use of paraprofessionals have been deficient. The accounts of Cleckley, Wagenfeld, and Riley et al., raise major questions regarding the usefulness of paraprofessionals.

Sections II and III of this volume raise the question: Why are paraprofessional programs in some areas more successful than in others? Before responding to this question, one must equivocate by noting, along with Blanton and Alley, that the assessment of success in a scientific manner is uncertain and infrequent for paraprofessional programs. The authors must also reiterate the political nature and use of some evaluations. If one stipulates, however, that the informal assessments and the analyses of expectations are substantially correct and the preponderance of evidence reported for given areas allow some conclusions, then one can address oneself to the question.

Part of the answer lies in the function served by the paraprofessional program. If the function is to save money by hiring less expensive paraprofessionals in lieu of more expensive professionals, then this is feasible virtually everywhere. If the purpose is to supply jobs for the unemployable or marginally employable this has been achieved with success. If, however, the purpose of the paraprofessional program is to provide a career ladder for the paraprofessional, or if the desired effect is to provide better services to clientele because of shared client-paraprofessional social identity and experiences, then the outcome is problematic. Finally, if the purpose of the paraprofessional program is to alter the structure of the service-providing organization and/or to change the roles, interaction patterns and power positions of the professional, then the outlook for success is dim. It seems clear to the authors that some of these functions are antithetical in given areas. If economies are sought in the hiring of paraprofessionals, then a large scale career ladder is inappropriate. If a bridge function is desired, then the restructuring of the caregiving network is an unlikely outcome. The greater the ambiguity of purpose for paraprofessionals, or the greater the number of functions desired of a paraprofessional program, the less likely it is to succeed.

Another part of the variability of paraprofessional assessment lies in the history of the area and the position of its professionals. In areas where service and structure are developed *de novo,* or where prior professional claim is absent, paraprofessional programs and activities may be very successful. The Home Start Program, a new concept in which professionals have never been involved, or the provision of mental health services on the Papago Reservation, where professional activity has not reached, are excellent examples of the success of paraprofessional programs. New tasks for paraprofessionals were not carved from the tasks of professionals or others already present in a functioning system. Questions of relative status and the problems of zero-sum relations of power need not be faced. Cleckley and Wagenfeld's analyses of the prarprofessionals' function in health and education and, to a lesser degree, Scott's comments on the use of paraprofessionals in corrections constitute examples of poorly faring paraprofessional programs because of latent and manifest contests with other members of the system for functions, power and resources. As seen in Wagenfeld's analysis of paraprofessionals in education, the situation can be exacerbated and the intention of the program thwarted when professional and paraprofessional compete in an arena of dwindling resources.

There is an additional consideration for the success of paraprofessionals. In order to serve the "bridgeman function," the paraprofessional must "represent" or "be of" the clientele in more than a general way. The ismorphism of the alcoholism counselor who may be a recovering alcoholic (the basis of AA) is great and the contribution of such a paraprofessional to the recovery of the alcoholic is different from, and in addition to, the contribution of the professional in the program. Similarly, the mental health paraprofessional on the Papago Reservation and the ex-offender corrections paraprofessional have valuable insights into the population being served. The bridge function of teacher aides, med techs, or nurses aides in a hospital may be based upon very flimsy, superficial similarities between clientele served and the paraprofessional.

It is instructive to analyze the state of paraprofessionalism as a social movement. The factors of proposed functions of paraprofessional programs, existing structure, and the history of areas in which the paraprofessional is introduced, as well as the precise convergence of paraprofessional and clientele characteristics, provide a basis with which to understand the variegated evaluations of paraprofessionals. This, in turn, leads the authors to a series of recommendations about the employment and support of paraprofessionals.

The authors began this concluding chapter by counterposing the positive and negative assessments of paraprofessionals: the movement could be regarded as either a dismal failure or a solid success that has become institutionalized as part of the fabric of the human services. The subsequent analysis indicated that neither polar view was entirely correct. One has to consider the movement in terms of the multiplicity of goals and functions envisaged for paraprofessionals as well as in terms of the large number of areas in which they were working.

What recommendations can be made to those responsible for the formulation and implementation of paraprofessional programs and the allocation of fiscal resources? The first point has less to do with specific programs and resources than it does with broader value questions. In her article, Cleckley questioned the advisability of using various categories of physician extenders in our health care system as a substitute for fully credentialed professionals. Without at all questioning the ability of these paraprofessionals to perform certain specific functions, the fact remains that they would likely be used differentially in the poorer sectors of our society: inner city and rural areas. Would this not, then, be formalizing or institutionalizing a two-tiered system of care? Although there would be a redress of some of the service delivery inequities, it would be at the cost of a certain parity. The use of paraprofessionals in situations like this would likely insure a minimum "floor" of services for all, but do essentially nothing to alter the greater access to high quality services available to the urban and the affluent. It should be clear that this policy issue is one created from ideology and values and, thus, not susceptible to empirical solutions. Whatever answer emerges is likely to be based on economic feasibility and political reality. The point, although directed toward the example of health care, nonetheless, has clear implications for the use of paraprofessionals in all of the human services. If providing minimum services at the risk of attenuating quality is acceptable because of the present paucity of services, then these types of paraprofessional programs should be supported.

A more specific recommendation involves a change of perspective. It is misleading to think of paraprofessionalism in some unitary fashion. Both the general overviews and the specific "state of the art" papers in this volume bring to mind the parable of the blind men attempting to describe an elephant. Programmatic and policy ends might better be served through selective and judicious deployment of resources in those areas of paraprofessional functioning in which there is the greatest likelihood of success. This is possible only after global efforts at generalization are abandoned.

This is not a call to eschew innovation. Rather, what is intended is a call for a more selective and specific approach to the area. Resources should be allocated to those innovative programs in which professional structures are either absent or from which professional activity is remote. High priority should be awarded paraprofessional programs in which paraprofessionals supply human services with which they, as individuals, have close personal experiences. When paraprofessional programs are contemplated in areas of high structure, strong professional presence and multiple goals, decisions should be made very cautiously. The problems these factors pose must be addressed and, hopefully, solved prior to the investment of monies, time, energy, and human hope. Since these conditions affecting the potential of paraprofessionals are visible, they should not be ignored in future planning and evaluation activities.

One of the most instructive aspects of Pearl's article for policy considerations in his vision of the future. For him, little of the institutional structure that was supposed to have been modified by paraprofessionals has, in fact, been changed. The kind of sustained political constituency necessary for change never existed. Paraprofessionals were created and imposed from above, more out of a sense of political expediency and a desire to pacify the poor, than out of a genuine concern for changing imporperly functioning social structures. What types of commitment are necessary on the part of society to bring about this basic change? For Pearl, it is nothing less than a radical shift away from our consumption-oriented industrial society to a human-services society. Only in such a new social order can the full potential of the paraprofessional's contributions be realized. Thus, his prescription for a better society involves substituting the changes paraprofessionals will make for society for the changes to be made in society for paraprofessionals (along with others). The picture that he paints of this new society has many appealing aspects. As a basis for social policy, however, it hardly seems likely to be adopted. Any social policy contains—either explicitly or implicitly—some cost-benefit calculus. Is the prevailing sentiment in our society supportive of this shift? Considering both the Proposition 13 mood and a notable unwillingness to make any meaningful lifestyle sacrifices that would result in energy savings, the answer is obvious. This perspective is inappropriate as a basis for paraprofessional policy making.

The concept of "social movement" seemed to be an appropriate frame of reference for considering some aspects of paraprofessionalism. One of the characteristics of social movements is that they progress through certain stages or phases. Early stages are characterized by an unfocused sense of discontent. Later, with the emergence of leaders and an ideology, the movement moves forward with a strong, often zealous, sense of mission. If the movement is successful, it is likely to become institutionalized —part of the social structure. The charismatic fervor of the early stages is replaced by a more bureaucratic orientation that is—quite appropriately concerned with issues of consolidation of gains and integration with the larger society. The early goals of the social movement are modified and partial goal attainment is substituted for the broader social change goals of an earlier time. This has been the case with paraprofessionalism. Currently, one does not hear the clarion calls to battle that were sounded in the late 1960s and early 1970s. With para-professionals solidly entrenched in many human services areas, concern has turned to issues such as organization and unionization. Even the name reflects this shift. Increasingly, the term "new professionals" is being used instead of "paraprofessional."

Policy makers, therefore, must recognize that the goals of the paraprofessional movement are not as they were at the earlier stages of the movement. The opportunity is present for a winnowing of the multiplicity of goals, a rectification of the goals so they are not functionally antithetical and a clarification and sharpening of the remaining goals. With this process completed, the support of paraprofessionalism and the investing of resources can be focused and paraprofessionalism applied for those purposes and to those areas where maximal contributions can be realized.

## REFERENCE NOTES

Riley, William. The Paraprofessional Polemic: Investigating the Case of the Paraprofessional in the Community Mental Health Center. Unpublished M.A. thesis, Western Michigan University, 1976.

## REFERENCES

Heberle, Rudolf *Social movements.* Appleton-Century-Crofts, Inc., New York, 1951.

McPherson, William *Ideology and change: Radicalism and fundamentalism in America.* National Press Books, Palo Alto: Calif., 1973.

Roberts, Ron E. and Robert Marsh Kloss *Social movements: Between the balcony and the barricade.* The C. V. Mosby Co., St. Louis, 1974.

Turner, Ralph and Lewis Killian *Collective behavior.* Prentice-Hall, Englewood Cliffs, N.J., 1972.

# Index

359

# Tolley's
# Tax Guide
# 2006–07

by

# Arnold Homer

# Rita Burrows

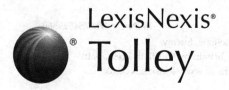

**Members of the LexisNexis Group worldwide**

| | |
|---|---|
| United Kingdom | LexisNexis Butterworths, a Division of Reed Elsevier (UK) Ltd, RSH, 1–3 Baxter's Place, Leith Walk, EDINBURGH EH1 3AF and Halsbury House, 35 Chancery Lane, LONDON WC2A 1EL |
| Argentina | LexisNexis Argentina, Buenos Aires |
| Australia | LexisNexis Butterworths, Chatswood, New South Wales |
| Austria | LexisNexis Verlag ARD Orac GmbH & Co KG, Vienna |
| Benelux | LexisNexis Benelux, Amsterdam |
| Canada | LexisNexis Canada, Markham, Ontario |
| Chile | LexisNexis Chile Ltda, Santiago |
| China | LexisNexis China, Beijing and Shanghai |
| France | LexisNexis SA, Paris |
| Germany | LexisNexis Deutschland GmbH, Munster |
| Hong Kong | LexisNexis Hong Kong, Hong Kong |
| India | LexisNexis India, New Delhi |
| Italy | Giuffrè Editore, Milan |
| Japan | LexisNexis Japan, Tokyo |
| Malaysia | Malayan Law Journal Sdn Bhd, Kuala Lumpur |
| Mexico | LexisNexis Mexico, Mexico |
| New Zealand | LexisNexis NZ Ltd, Wellington |
| Poland | Wydawnictwo Prawnicze LexisNexis Sp, Warsaw |
| Singapore | LexisNexis Singapore, Singapore |
| South Africa | LexisNexis Butterworths, Durban |
| USA | LexisNexis, Dayton, Ohio |

© Reed Elsevier (UK) Ltd 2006

Published by LexisNexis Butterworths

A CIP Catalogue record for this book is available from the British Library.

[Twenty-fifth edition]

ISBN 10: 0754529568                     ISBN 13: 9780754529569

Typeset by Letterpart Ltd, Reigate, Surrey

Printed and bound in Great Britain by CPI Bath Press, Bath

Visit LexisNexis Butterworths at www.lexisnexis.co.uk